Education Policy

~~TWO~~ WEEK LOAN

In this up-to-date introduction to a key policy area, Paul Trowler puts current education policy into context by showing how it has evolved over time and in response to different political ideals. He examines what education policy is, how it is formulated and, crucially, how the processes of implementation affect outcomes. He looks at the key issues facing the government today and at how the research process feeds into policy-making. This concise guide is suitable for both students and professionals and features:

- policy landmark tables
- illustrative case studies
- summaries of key points
- guides to further reading
- useful websites and addresses
- a glossary of key terms

Paul Trowler is Reader in Higher Education, Lancaster University.

The Gildredge Social Policy Series provides introductory textbooks to key areas of policy for the growing number of students of social policy at A level, A/S level, on GNVQ courses, in their first year at university or following a professional diploma course. Written by experienced teachers, the books are short, tightly structured texts designed to be aids to learning.

Series editor: **Pete Alcock**, Professor of Social Policy and Administration, University of Birmingham.

Also in this series:

Education Policy

Second edition

Paul Trowler

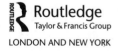

Routledge
Taylor & Francis Group

LONDON AND NEW YORK

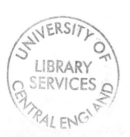

First published 1998
Second edition 2003
by Routledge
11 New Fetter Lane, London EC4P 4EE

Simultaneously published in the USA and Canada
by Routledge
29 West 35th Street, New York, NY 10001

Routledge is an imprint of the Taylor & Francis Group

© 1998, 2003 Paul Trowler

Typeset in Times by
Keystroke, Jacaranda Lodge, Wolverhampton

Printed and bound in Great Britain by
Biddles Ltd, Guildford and King's Lynn

British Library Cataloguing in Publication Data
A catalogue record for this book is available from the British Library

Library of Congress Cataloging in Publication Data
Trowler, Paul.
  Education policy / Paul Trowler.–2nd ed.
    p. cm. – (Gildredge social policy series)
  Includes bibliographical references (p.) and index.
  1. Education and state–Great Britain. I. Title. II. Series.

LC93.G7 T658 2002
379.41–dc21   2002068243

ISBN 0–415–27553–9 (hbk)
ISBN 0–415–27554–7 (pbk)

Contents

Tables and figures

Tables

Figures

Foreword

This book seeks to present the background to education policy for the novice or near-novice reader, contextualizing it in a theoretical understanding of how policy is made and the processes involved in its implementation. Ball and Shilling (1994, p. 1) have noted that this field has given rise to large numbers of concepts, often dislocated from contexts or explanatory frameworks. This book seeks to locate important concepts in a series of case studies for you, so that their application can be understood. You should bear in mind, however, that in every field of social science concepts tend to shift in their meaning both over time and according to context.

The structure of the book is as follows. Chapters 1 and 2 set out the historical background to education policy in the compulsory and post-compulsory sectors respectively, and each presents case studies to allow the exploration of some important policy issues in more depth. Chapter 3 seeks to give insight into how education policy is made and into some of the influences on the policy formulation process. Chapter 4 looks at the important questions of how policy is received on the ground, how it is implemented and the significance of this for outcomes. For clarity I have used the traditional language of 'policy-making' and 'policy implementation', with its implication that these are distinct phases in the policy process. Again, you should be aware that 'policy-making' happens at a number of points in the policy process, including at the point of putting it into effect. Chapter 5 examines some key issues for education policy that face governments. Finally, Chapter 6 considers the relationship between education research and education policy. The Glossary explains at least some of the terms which may be new to a novice reader. Most chapters contain a list of useful addresses and websites, as well as suggestions for further reading. These websites were operational at the time of going to press but because of the nature of the World Wide Web they may move to new addresses or no longer be in operation. Updates to them, information on current education policy and links to new relevant websites can be found at: http://www.lancs.ac.uk/staff/trowler. The book was first published in 1998. For the 2003 edition I have updated some of the readings and the website addresses and included the latest information about policy developments which occurred during the Labour government's 1997–2001 term of office. The book attempts to discuss the education system across the whole of the UK. However, this has not always been possible both for reasons of space and because the education systems in the four countries of the UK have become increasingly diversified with the effects of devolution of government. England, or England and Wales together, probably receive more attention than Scotland and Northern Ireland here, though where there are very significant differences these have been identified.

Having read the book you should:

- understand the nature of education policy
- appreciate the processes involved in education policy-making and the important factors which impinge on them
- understand the ways in which the policy implementation process can lead to an 'implementation gap' between what is intended by policy-makers and what actually happens
- have a grounding in policies in both compulsory and post-compulsory education, particularly those put into effect since 1979
- be aware of important contemporary issues in education policy
- appreciate important links between policy and education research, as well as understanding the reasons for the often tenuous nature of those links.

In short, having read the book, you should be able to understand, interpret and discuss educational policies in a more sophisticated way. I hope you enjoy it too.

Paul Trowler
Lancaster University, March 2002

Chapter 1
Policies and structures
Schools

OUTLINE
This chapter first outlines the background to the present system of compulsory education in the UK. It then goes on to give a summary of the landmarks in formal education policy on schools between 1979 (the year of the Conservatives' election to government) and 2001. An overview of the situation in 1997, when the Labour government was first elected, and then in 2001, is provided together with a discussion of education policy-making during the eighteen years of Conservative administration prior to that. A case study of one of the key aspects of education policy during that period is provided, namely parental choice of schools, and through it some of the important aspects of New Right educational ideas are explored. The chapter concludes with a summary of key points covered. It is important to note that, while this chapter and Chapter 2 concentrate on legislative and other formal policy events, subsequent chapters go on to show that policy should be conceived in broader terms than simply the formal actions of government and other official agencies.

Background to the current system

Before 1870 the role of the state in education was limited to the provision of grants to some church schools, some teacher training responsibility and the education of pauper children in schools associated with some workhouses. Church, private and voluntary schools were the only important sources of education. Only the middle class and the upper class could afford an education of any quality, and this was usually limited to their male children.

The 1870 (Forster's) Elementary Education Act set up elected authorities, School Boards, to establish schools where existing provision was inadequate. These were funded from the rates, and education was made available for 5 to 13 year olds, although it was not compulsory. Compulsory education to the age of 10 years was introduced in 1880; fees for elementary education for most children were abolished in 1891, allowing the further extension of the school leaving age. This was extended to 11 years in 1893 and 12 years in 1899. In 1893 it became compulsory for school authorities to make provision for blind and deaf children up to the age of 16 years.

The 1902 (Balfour's) Education Act made local authorities rather than School Boards responsible for schools, including church schools. The basis of today's organization of education, run by local authorities, was thus laid. The County Councils and County Borough Councils had been created in 1888 under the Local Government Act.

The 1918 Education Act raised the school leaving age to 14 years. Increasing national control of education was established, with central government also accepting more of the burden of cost. Local authorities had now to report to a central Board of Education.

Free secondary education for all

Butler's 1944 Education Act was based on three reports:

* The 1926 Hadow Report recommended increasing the school leaving age to 15 years, selective secondary education beginning at 11 years and parity of esteem – equal status – for different types of school.
* The 1938 Spens Report recommended a diversification of types of secondary schools.
* The 1943 Norwood Report recommended the tripartite system: the division into what would become the grammar, secondary modern and secondary technical schools.

The 1944 Act ensured compulsory and free state education from 5 to 15 years, and set up the primary (5–11 years), secondary (11–15 years) and further (16–18-plus) schools and colleges. It also marked the introduction of the tripartite system of education: the grammar, secondary modern and secondary technical schools, although few of the last were built. The goals were parity of esteem and easy transfer between the three types of schools, but neither was achieved.

However, the system set up by the Butler Act soon ran into criticism. The selection process, the 11-plus examination, was shown to be inefficient and biased towards the middle class. Four postwar reports on schools were very critical of the education system of the time.

The 1954 Gurney-Dixon Report (*Early Leaving*) looked at the factors which prevented children from staying at school beyond the statutory leaving age. It concluded that pupils' performance, and their likelihood of staying on at school, was strongly linked to parental social class. The Report offered some ideas about why this should be the case; it cast serious doubt upon the extent to which the 1944 Act had achieved its stated aim of establishing a meritocratic system in which a child's potential was identified and nurtured in appropriate circumstances.

The 1959 Crowther Report (*Fifteen to Eighteen*) pointed out that most 15–18 year olds received no formal education despite the expansion of courses in further education and technical colleges. The Report recommended that there should be more further education to prevent the wastage of talent of those who left school at 15 years to follow a craft or technical career. It also recommended the raising of the school leaving age to 16 years.

The 1963 Newsom Report (*Half Our Future*) found that accommodation was deficient in 80 per cent of schools attended by average and below-average ability students. These were mainly secondary modern schools. While not disagreeing with the tripartite system, it recommended more spending on secondary modern schools in slum areas. Newsom confirmed the Crowther recommendation for the raising of the school leaving age.

Finally the 1967 Plowden Report (*Children and Their Primary Schools*) pointed out the deficiencies in schools in poorer areas. These included noisy environments, high staff turnover, inadequate facilities and large class sizes. The Report recommended positive discrimination for schools in deprived areas, which would be termed Educational Priority Areas (EPAs). Extra money was to be made available for better staff–pupil ratios and facilities. Suggestions were also made to improve school management, to abolish corporal punishment and to appoint specialists to look into the particular problems found in these schools.

The move to comprehensive schools

The election of a Labour government under Prime Minister Harold Wilson in 1964 marked a turn in central government's attitude towards the tripartite system. The Ministry of Education issued Circular 10/65 asking all local education authorities (LEAs) to submit plans for a reorganization of the tripartite into a comprehensive system. This is a system of non-selective schools which accept all children from their catchment area. Already in 1962 one secondary school pupil in ten was in a comprehensive or near-comprehensive school. In 1964 71 per cent of all LEAs had or intended to have some form of comprehensivization in their area. Circular 10/65 was consolidating a trend which had begun locally in the 1950s. By 1982 well over 80 per cent of secondary school pupils were in comprehensive schools. This was despite the Conservative Party's hostility to comprehensives and, upon being elected to government in 1970, its issuing of Circular 10/70 recommending the re-establishment of selectivity.

The 1970 Education Act improved provision for children with disabilities and learning difficulties. In 1972 the school leaving age was raised to 16 years. A Labour government was returned in 1974; its 1976 Education Act imposed a non-selective system on all LEAs, although some refused to implement it. (This Act was repealed by the 1979 Education Act.)

The origin of the new vocationalism

In 1976 the Labour Prime Minister James Callaghan gave his famous Ruskin speech, at Ruskin College Oxford. Amongst other things he said:

> I am concerned in my journeys to find complaints from industry that new recruits from schools sometimes do not have the basic tools to do the job that is required [and] . . . that many

of our best trained students who have completed the higher levels of education at university or polytechnic have no desire or intention of joining industry . . . The goals of our education, from nursery school through to adult education, are clear enough. They are to equip children to the best of their ability for a lively, constructive place in society and also to fit them to do a job of work. Not one or the other, but both . . . The balance was wrong in the past. We have a responsibility now in this generation to see that we do not get it wrong in the other direction . . . Both of the basic purposes of education require the same essential tools. These are to be basically literate, to be basically numerate, to understand how to live and work together, to have respect for others and respect for the individual.

(Callaghan 1976, pp. 10–16)

This speech was the keynote for education policy that would follow, particularly in the eighteen years of Conservative government that were to begin only three years after Callaghan made that speech. Callaghan's articulation of these ideas publicly at this time marked, essentially, the end of the Butskellite consensus (see Glossary) and a new ideological underpinning for education policy-making.

The situation in 1997

Pre-primary school education

Over 90 per cent of 3 and 4 year olds received some form of pre-primary provision. About a quarter went to state (maintained) nursery schools and classes, another quarter to infant classes in maintained primary schools and the bulk of the rest went to privately run playgroups.

Compulsory education

Most areas had a two-tier system in which pupils changed from primary to secondary school at around the age of 11 years. Most areas had comprehensive secondary education, although some

Table 1.1 Compulsory education policy: some landmarks since 1979

Key policy events	Selected key content	Commentary
1979 Education Act	Repealed the obligation on LEAs to make plans for comprehensivization of secondary schools.	The Conservatives' opposition to the comprehensive principle is demonstrated by this very rapid legislation, repealing the Labour government's 1976 Act.
1980 Education Act	• Assisted places scheme put in place. • Parents given right to choose the school they wanted (though LEAs could refuse on grounds of inefficient use of resources). • Parents given rights to be represented on school governing bodies. • School governors required to provide information to parents on a variety of matters (exam results, criteria for admission, curriculum etc.). • Restricted certain powers of LEAs and gave Education Secretary more powers in certain areas of policy.	This Act sets the foundations for Conservative legislation on education in the years to come. Assisted places allowed 'bright' pupils from the maintained education sector to transfer to private schools with all or part of their fees paid by government. In the eyes of critics this scheme demonstrated the government's view that maintained schools were not good enough to cater for bright pupils and its lack of determination to improve them. The rights and powers given to parents and to governors mark the initiation of a series of policy measures designed, on the one hand, to introduce market rigours to the education service by empowering parents as consumers and, on the other, empowering schools (rather than LEAs) to take action to compete in a market

		environment. Essentially this Act and later ones was predicated on the idea of shifting the balance of power in the education system towards parents and individual schools and away from LEAs and shifting the nature of the system away from a 'command' (planned, directed) towards a 'market' one.
1981 Education Act	■ Gave LEAs responsibilities to define the needs of special needs children and determine appropriate provision. ■ Affirmed the idea of 'mainstreaming' special needs children (i.e. teaching them in ordinary schools where possible). ■ Gave parents of special needs children the right to be consulted on and to appeal against decisions concerning their child.	Largely implemented the recommendations of the 1978 Warnock Report, particularly the idea of mainstreaming and 'statementing' special needs children. A statement is a report drawn up by a multi-disciplinary team concerning the nature of a child's special needs and how best to address them.
1982 Announcement of the Technical and Vocational Education Initiative (TVEI) by Margaret Thatcher	Pilot schemes set up in 1983 by the Manpower Services Commission (MSC). TVEI would run for over ten years. Its aims were: ■ to focus on and improve technical and vocational education for 14–18 year olds in schools and colleges ■ to include planned work experience ■ full-time programmes to be delivered which combined general and technical and vocational education.	Initial doubts and uncertainties among LEAs, schools and colleges began to disappear as it became clear that locally it was possible to develop and control TVEI projects and that they brought useful sums of money. Local TVEI co-ordinators and their steering groups remained in control. By the mid-1980s TVEI involved most LEAs and provided 'unprecedentedly large amounts of money for those involved' (Dale 1985b, p. 44). When it wound down in the early 1990s it

continued

Table 1.1 *continued*

Key policy events	Selected key content	Commentary
1982 Announcement of the Technical and Vocational Education Initiative (TVEI) by Margaret Thatcher (continued)	TVEI was split up into a number of local projects rather than run as a centrally directed scheme. The projects were to be carefully monitored to establish good practice for the whole ability range.	was widely considered to have been a success and early fears that it would excessively vocationalize the curriculum proved unfounded. Around 1.3 million 14–18 year olds participated in TVEI in 1993/4, roughly 78% of the total population of that age.

Dale (1985b) notes the unusual features of TVEI:

■ Its genesis was unusual: there was no consultation, no legislation and no committee of enquiry: Margaret Thatcher surprised everyone when she announced it. It was introduced into education from outside.

■ It was bigger and more extensive than most other education initiatives.

■ It represented an obvious break with what had gone before and was introduced at tremendous speed with very ambitious goals.

■ Project management, finances and other aspects of TVEI were outside the normal patterns: for example the steering groups were outside the normal LEA management structures.

1985 White Paper *Better Schools*	Stated that the government would not assume greater powers over the school curriculum.	Written while Keith Joseph, one of the leaders of the neo-liberal faction of the New Right (see p. 104), was education secretary, this was later to become something of an embarrassment as the government was only three years later to set up the national curriculum, and a range of other legislation gave strong powers to the Secretary of State for Education. This illustrates the way policy does not necessarily advance incrementally but is subject to negotiation, compromise and hence change.
1986 Education Act (there were two, but only one is of interest here)	■ Set out a formula by which the composition of the governing body of every maintained (LEA) school is calculated: determining how many parents, voluntary body and LEA representatives should be included. ■ Increased parent representation on governing bodies. ■ Required more information to be given by governors to parents, for example detailed annual reports.	Built on the foundations laid by the 1980 Act to give parents more control over schools and to ensure that parents as consumers of education should have adequate information on which to base their decisions. Prepared the ground for later legislation by firming up the structure and role of school governing bodies.

continued

Table 1.1 *continued*

Key policy events	Selected key content	Commentary
1988 Higginson Report	A committee set up by the government under Dr Gordon Higginson to look at education in the 16–18 age range. The committee considered that the education provided by the current A level system was too narrow: students specialized too early and it should be broadened to become more like the French Baccalaureate. Specifically a five subject structure was proposed.	This subject has has stimulated political controversy and continues to do so. On the one hand the argument runs that the A level system is too narrow and specialized for the needs of a modern economy. On the other the A level is regarded as the 'gold standard' which underpins the quality of education above and below it. The Higginson proposals were rejected. Margaret Thatcher favoured the A level 'gold standard'. However the idea proved popular in some education circles and it was given fresh impetus by the publication in 1990 of the paper 'A British Baccalaureate' (Finegold et al.), one co-author of which was David Miliband, who was to become chief policy adviser to Tony Blair in 1997 and school minister in 2002.
1988 Education Act	■ Gave the Education Secretary powers to prescribe a national curriculum for pupils to the age of 16 in maintained schools. ■ Set up the National Curriculum Council (for England) to oversee the content and assessment of the national curriculum.	The most important Education Act concerning schools since 1944. This further extended the idea of 'parental choice' of schools both by reducing the powers of the LEAs to restrict where children go (they could now go to any maintained school that

- Gave greater freedom for parents to select the maintained school of their choice.
- Ensured that maintained schools should not artificially limit the number of pupils. It did this by setting the normal school roll as that of 1979 (when rolls were at their highest).
- LEAs required to delegate 'hiring and firing' of school staff to schools' governing bodies.
- Set up mechanisms for schools to opt out of LEA control to become grant-maintained (GM) schools if the majority of parents who voted in a secret ballot desired this.
- Set up the mechanisms for the establishment of City Technology Colleges (CTCs).
- Staff appraisal schemes made a legal requirement.

had room for them provided it catered for their age and aptitude). Again, this built on earlier Acts. Now, however, the idea of extending the options available to parents was given greater force by the plans to permit grant-maintained (GM) schools, which were more or less self-governing (i.e. free of LEA control), and the city technology colleges, which were designed to have more of an emphasis on technology, languages and business and commerce than other types of schools. By 1995 there were around a thousand GM schools. They must implement the national curriculum and are subject to OFSTED inspection (see below).

Even maintained schools which did not want or achieve GM status would now have greater powers to control their own affairs under this Act, a position usually referred to as LMS: local management of schools. Schools, or at least their governing bodies, now had more power to control their own financial affairs and to hire and fire staff. Conversely the role and powers of the LEAs, already weakened by earlier legislation, were further reduced.

continued

Table 1.1 *continued*

Key policy events	Selected key content	Commentary
1988 Education Act (continued)		This reflected a fundamental animosity towards LEAs on the part of central government. They were seen as self-interested, overblown, inefficient and expensive bureaucracies. Moreover, during a period in which the Conservative government had a large majority in Parliament and, in the main, the support of the House of Lords, local government in general was the only stronghold of opposition. Much of local government, and therefore LEAs, was in Labour hands at the time.
		It is worth noting the way in which this Act contains strong elements of dirigisme: directing education from the centre (e.g. through the national curriculum) and market liberalism (e.g. through setting up different 'flavours' of schools). In this it was reflecting the tension between neo-conservatism and neo-liberalism in New Right thinking. Chapter 3 addresses this issue in more detail as well as giving background information on the policy processes underpinning the development of the national curriculum and GM schools policy.

| 1992 The 'Three Wise Men' report published: *Curriculum Organization and Classroom Practice in Primary Schools* (see page 178–9). | The authors were tasked to 'review available evidence about the delivery of education in primary schools' and to 'make recommendations about curriculum organization, teaching methods and classroom practice appropriate for the successful implementation of the National Curriculum, particularly at Key Stage 2'. | Widely interpreted as an attack on 'progressivist' methods of teaching in primary schools and a call for a return to whole-class didactic teaching of subjects, not topics, the reception of this leant weight to the traditionalist educational viewpoint and the New Right attack on 'progressivism' in schools. |
| 1992 Education (Schools) Act | ■ Set up new school inspection arrangements by establishing the Office for Standards in Education (OFSTED), a department independent of the DfEE and, in England, under the direction of Her Majesty's Chief Inspector of Schools – currently (2002) Mike Tomlinson.

■ OFSTED was charged with identifying, training and registering teams of school inspectors, under a registered inspector ('regie') who will go into schools (once every four years in theory) for around a week and write a publicly available report. | This Act demonstrates the neo-liberal strand of Conservative thinking (see p. 104). Instead of the official body of Her Majesty's Inspectors (HMI) who previously inspected schools and wrote private reports, school inspection is effectively privatized. Inspection teams, once trained and registered, now bid for a contract to inspect schools, thus imposing some market discipline in terms of cost, efficiency and effectiveness (in theory). The teams must include at least one lay inspector (not involved professionally with education), thus opening up what was previously seen as a professional 'closed shop' (the Conservative government felt that the HMI had been in the pockets of the teaching profession: an example of 'producer capture' |

continued

Table 1.1 *continued*

Key policy events	Selected key content	Commentary
1992 Education (Schools) Act (continued)		in which those who provide a service control and run it in their own interests, not those of the consumer). Reports are publicly available in libraries, on the World Wide Web and elsewhere, thus empowering the parent as consumer with the data they need to make informed choices. (See the end of this chapter for the OFSTED website address.)
1993 Dearing Report	This government-appointed review into the national curriculum recommended that: ■ the curriculum should be slimmed down ■ the time given to testing should be reduced ■ around 20% of teaching time should be freed up for use at the discretion of schools ■ for Key Stage 4 (i.e. 14–16 years) the school's discretion should be extended even further, with art, geography, history and music made optional ■ curriculum choice at Key Stage 3 ■ National Curriculum Council (NCC) and Schools Examination and Assessment Council (SEAC) should become one body: the Schools Assessment Authority (SCAA).	The government accepted Dearing's recommendations. Subsequent changes to the national curriculum cost £744 million. It had by this time become clear that the national curriculum had grown into an unwieldy structure which was almost impossible to implement and which was proving in some cases detrimental to good teaching and learning because teachers' time was increasingly being spent on paperwork and testing rather than teaching. The Dearing Report gave the government an opportunity to try to improve the curriculum and its associated tests without losing too much face.

1993 Education Act	
■ Set up the Funding Agency for Schools (FAS) which would finance GM schools.	This 'tidied up' a number of features put in place by earlier policies and took even further
■ FAS also directed to eventually take over some of the powers of LEAs to plan provision in their areas.	the erosion of powers of the LEAs, which by now were becoming worried about their future role in education (Morris et al., 1993).
■ Simplified 'opting out' procedures for schools to become GM.	
■ Introduced methods to deal with 'failing schools' when these were so identified by OFSTED inspectors.	
■ National Curriculum Council and School Examinations and Assessment Council replaced by a single School Curriculum and Assessment Authority.	

1994 Education Act	
■ Established the Teacher Training Agency (TTA) for England and Wales.	Widely seen in the university sector as a threat to their control over the provision of teacher
■ The TTA funds teacher training in England and promotes teaching as a career.	training, this policy was designed to make teacher education more 'practical' and less 'theoretical'. This was based partly on
■ Schools are to be centrally involved in delivering courses for initial and in-service education and training of teachers and managers. This may be on their own or in partnership with others, including with higher education institutions.	government distrust of teacher educators in higher education and partly on a desire to tackle the supposed problems within schools (such as those addressed by the 'Three Wise Men' report) at their roots.

continued

Table 1.1 continued

Key policy events	Selected key content	Commentary
1996 Nursery Education and Grant Maintained Schools Act	■ Extended nursery vouchers to the whole nation from April 1997. ■ Enabled schools to borrow from commercial markets for capital projects.	The nursery vouchers aspect of this would be the first of the Conservative education policies to be axed by the incoming Labour government in 1997. Plans were also quickly developed by Labour to change the nature and funding of GM schools, set out in the White Paper *Excellence in Schools* (see Chapter 5). The provisions of the 1996 Act, then, were extremely short lived.
1996 Changes to school inspections announced and the new *Framework* and *Handbook for School Inspection in England* published	■ School inspections to become more manageable and less bureaucratic. ■ Sharper focus on standards and teaching. ■ For inspectors less form-filling; fewer but more explicit criteria on which to assess performance. ■ Better format for small primary and nursery schools. ■ Judgements to be expressed more clearly and in a more focused way.	This was designed to rectify some of the unintended consequences of the new system of inspection which had become apparent. These are vividly illustrated in a quotation from a researcher studying the effects of inspection in one school: 'I am moved by the pain of it all, by the stress, by the plummeting of self esteem, by seeing how their cherished values in terms of pedagogy are being marginalized, by the fear of failure, and by the tensions created. I am particularly moved by the way in which these people who have committed themselves to

their pupils and their work, and gained over the years some measure of confidence about what they do and can contribute to society, find themselves as no more than units to be examined and observed, scrutinized and assessed. This particular week was the lowest time for them as they entered into the fringes of the central spotlight of power – the OFSTED inspection' (Woods 1996, p. 102).

1997 Education Act

- Allowed GM schools to expand.
- Enabled schools to be more selective without having to gain central approval to do so.
- Permitted exclusions of pupils for up to 45 days.
- Children to be tested upon entry to primary school.
- OFSTED given powers to inspect LEAs.
- Assisted places scheme extended to prep schools (40 institutions).
- New Qualifications and Curriculum Authority (QCA) set up to combine NCVQ (see p. 203) and SCAA (see p. 203).

The last piece of Conservative government education legislation before the general election of May 1997. Labour would initially leave the OFSTED powers in place, believing that LEAs had to prove they added value to educational provision and that the principle of 'zero tolerance of failure' should apply to them too. The QCA came into existence and the testing of children on admission also came into effect, as did the provisions on the exclusion of pupils. Other measures were quickly changed by Labour, however (see Chapter 5).

continued

Table 1.1 *continued*

Key policy events	Selected key content	Commentary
1997 The new Labour government publishes *Excellence in Schools* White Paper	This White Paper announced the following: ■ setting up of a Standards Task Force ■ instituting a Standards and Efficiency unit at the DfEE ■ setting a target for 2002 of 80% of all 11 year olds to reach the required standard of literacy and 75% to reach the required standard of numeracy ■ requirement on all schools to establish challenging targets for themselves in their development plans, and LEAs to do likewise ■ introduction of General Teaching Council to represent the education profession ■ creation of posts for advanced skills teachers ■ funding for more and better in-service training for teachers who have shown special abilities and can act as models of excellence ■ policies for valuing teachers and celebrating good practice and excellence ■ developing a new curriculum for initial teacher training	*Excellence in Schools* was based on six key principles: ■ Education is at the heart of government. ■ Education should be for the benefit of the many, not the few. ■ Standards, not structures and institutions, need to change. ■ Intervention in what is wrong, not what is working well. ■ Zero tolerance of failure. ■ Commitment to work in partnership with all interested parties. These marked a clear change from what had gone before, at least in terms of rhetoric. The incoming Labour government declared that its three priorities for government would be 'education, education, education' and this refrain was repeated in the months after the election (Blair 1997). The first Labour budget, in July 1997, allocated a total of £2.3 billion of extra resources for schools in the UK: £1.3 billion on capital spending and £1 billion on revenue. In education policy, as in other

areas, Labour insisted it would be 'firm but fair', providing resources where needed but requiring results in the form of improved standards. Meanwhile the Labour government's Welfare to Work programme meant that 18–24 year olds would have only one of the following options: take up a job; do a six-month placement with the Environment Task Force or an organization in the voluntary sector, or become a full-time student. Refusal to take one of these options would mean loss of benefit. This policy on unemployment and benefits promised to have important knock-on consequences for post-compulsory education with a potential flood of new (and under-qualified) students moving into colleges and universities.

- making qualifications for head teachers mandatory
- establishment of education action zones which give additional support for struggling schools, usually in inner-city areas
- a policy to establish a 'national grid for learning': an internet system for schools and phasing out of GM schools and introduction of a new system in which schools fall into one of three categories: aided, community or foundation schools
- allocation of more seats to parents on governing bodies
- allowing parents to decide the future of grammar schools.

November 1997 *Connecting the Learning Society: National Grid for Learning* published

Set out plans for information and communication technology (ICT) revolution in schools:

- All schools and colleges to be connected to the internet by 1998. Full implementation of plan set out in this paper by 2002.
- Technology to be used for management information and teacher preparation as well as learning.

Here the new Labour government set out its plans to modernize the education system, bringing to it the benefits of ICT that had already been realized by commerce and industry. Although the White Paper recognizes the formidable task of bringing teachers up to date with this technology, the more subtle implementation and teaching and learning issues are not addressed here.

continued

Table 1.1 *continued*

Key policy events	Selected key content	Commentary
November 1997 *Connecting the Learning Society: National Grid for Learning* published (continued)	■ Students to be able to find and download information to help them in their studies. ■ Government to encourage development of appropriate software as well as funding hardware links. ■ Teacher education to be acknowledged as an important task.	In some cases the use of ICT is not an appropriate tool for teaching and learning and has unwanted effects if used wrongly (e.g. loss of face-to-face interaction). Many teachers are not only unskilled in the use of ICT, they are quite strongly opposed to its use in the educative process. Pupils and students have a tendency to subvert the intended uses of technology and to use it for games, illicit communication and other purposes not intended, or approved of, by teachers and policy-makers.
School Standards and Framework Act (1998)	■ Class sizes to be thirty maximum for infants. ■ Education Action Zones to be run by local authorities and business – raising standards is the aim. ■ LEAs to draw up education development plans and early years development plans and have statutory duty to raise standards. ■ Government to have powers to take over failing LEAs.	Gibson and Asthana (1998) in their critique of this White Paper note that it appears to mark a 'rediscovery' of the importance of social background and structured patterns of social advantage or disadvantage in affecting the performance of schools. However, they note that the concept of Education Action Zones is 'extremely limited, both in scope and ambition' (p. 205). The focus of the programme is too narrow and the resources directed to it inadequate to address the scale

of disadvantage that needs to be addressed. However, the main difficulty which these and other critics identify with this thrust of policy is the fact that it is expects individual schools to address patterns of social disadvantage when the evidence is that schooling predominantly operates to reflect, even reinforce, patterns of advantage and disadvantage.

- Secretary of State to be able to shut failing schools and reopen with new head, new name and many new staff.
- Code of practice defining roles and responsibilities of LEAs to be introduced.
- Abolition of GM schools, new framework of community, voluntary and foundation schools put in place (heralded in *Excellence in Schools* White Paper).
- More parents on governing bodies and LEA committees.
- Ballots for local parents to abolish grammar school status.
- Adjudicator for admissions and schools reorganization to be appointed.
- Partial selection allowed to continue where it exists.
- Specialist schools to be allowed 10% selection by aptitude.
- Regulations on nutritional standards for school lunches.
- Duty for local authority to provide nursery education.
- Abolition of FAS.
- LEAs banned from setting up assisted-places-style schemes.

(See the *Times Educational Supplement* 13 March 1998 for more details.)

continued

Table 1.1 *continued*

Key policy events	Selected key content	Commentary
National Literacy Strategy published, March 1998	Sets out the programme of teaching literacy in primary schools for the next five years.	This development can be interpreted as another attack on teachers' claims to professional status or an enhancement of it.
	Details the amount of time to spent and what is to be done in very specific terms.	The 'deprofessionalization' argument runs like this: there has been a gradual de-skilling of teachers in Britain and abroad. Particularly identifiable has been a separation of conception from execution (Apple 1989). The national curriculum has told teachers *what* to teach, *when* to teach it and *how to test* what they have taught. The books and materials which support the national curriculum have taken the imaginative work of teaching away from them. Now, at last, central government is telling them not just *what* to teach, but *how* to teach it. The process of turning teachers into technicians continues.
	Those involved in literacy education will be trained in the prescribed approaches – this will take about two days per person.	
		The 'extended professionalization' argument runs that teaching is increasingly becoming an evidence-based profession with skilled practitioners using proven techniques,

rigorously evaluated and assessed, to achieve the best results. Professor Michael Barber says of the National Literacy Strategy: 'Here's the best practice, based on solid international research and experience', while the DfEE says 'this is the first time that every primary teacher in the country will understand and use best practice' (quoted Ghouri 1998). The supporters of the extended professionalization argument suggest that teachers will be enabled to become more creative and professional. The critics argue that this is a blueprint that will not apply in many situations: teaching is about using professional judgements in specific contexts, about being a 'reflective practitioner', and that the notion of proven universal solutions is simplistic and unworkable in educational contexts. (See Hammersley and Scarth 1993.)

June 1998 The setting up of twenty-five Action Zones announced for England: first twelve to be operational at the beginning of the new academic year. 140,000 pupils will eventually be educated in an Action Zone and Action Zones are targeted at some of the most deprived areas

■ £1 million per year being spent.
■ Each zone to have around twenty schools, primary and secondary.
■ A number of 'stakeholders' involved in the running of each zone: LEAs, business etc.
■ Zones expected to develop and implement innovative educational ideas which will spread through the system.

The big carrot is the funding which the Action Zones will attract. Certainly the zones represent a real attempt to tackle social disadvantage and to create equality of opportunity. In total around £56 million will be spent on around 140,000 of the children who most need it. However, concerns about the zones include the following points:

■ They represent the privatization of education by the back door.

continued

Table 1.1 *continued*

Key policy events	Selected key content	Commentary
National Literacy Strategy published, March 1998 (continued)	■ These to include, for example, specialist teachers; new curriculum ideas; better use of ICT; improved pupil records; extended school days and improved management.	■ Business will have too great a hand over children's education. ■ There is a contradiction between devolution of power to schools and control of schools within Action Zones. ■ The financial contribution from business has been too limited.
July 1998 Announcement of the Government's Comprehensive Spending Review outcomes	£19 billion extra for education in total: £3 billion in 1999; £6 billion in 2000; £10 billion in 2001.	The extra resources for education were welcomed by those in the education system and saw a shift towards increasing the share of the GDP devoted to education after some years of decline.
Teaching and Higher Education Act 1998	Though primarily to do with higher education, there are some provisions which relate to compulsory education. See p. 67 for a summary and commentary.	
23 March 1999 Government announces a three-year £350 million allocation for inner-city schools	This involved: ■ extra tuition to be available for the most able children – initially, 100,000 pupils in 450 schools in London, Manchester, Liverpool, Birmingham, Leeds, Bradford, Sheffield and Rotherham	Welcome focusing on needs of inner-city schools but assumption that schools can tackle the problems of society. Also rather strange that so much of this money is focused on higher achievers.

March 1999 Government announces outcome of *Qualifying for Success* consultation. 'The government believes that the traditional post-16 curriculum in England is too narrow and inflexible in the modern world' (letter from DfEE to educational institutions, 19 March 1999)

- the appointment of 800 'learning mentors' to work in the 450 target schools. These were designed to help underachievers make the most of educational opportunities – especially children from minority, ethnic and disadvantaged backgrounds.
- more 'learning units' for disruptive youngsters, to serve each of the 450 target schools.

This involves:

- new AS qualification (Advanced Subsidiary) to be equivalent to the first half of a full A level
- a new broader A level syllabus
- new 'synoptic' assessment at A level
- limits on amount of assessment by coursework
- new higher level tests to be more accessible than current S levels
- revisions to GNVQ
- separate certification of 'key skills' in GNVQ
- new key skills qualification.

The aim here is to broaden the 'too-narrow' education beyond 16 and to bring the UK into line with other countries. Wider skills acquisition is an important aim too.

continued

Table 1.1 *continued*

Key policy events	Selected key content	Commentary
March 1999 Green Paper: *Teachers – Meeting the Challenge of Change* published	■ All teachers to be appraised by senior staff. ■ Pay scales and teachers' career development to be determined by outcomes. ■ Teachers must prepare a portfolio providing information about their performance, analysis of pupils' results and evidence of commitment to their own professional development. ■ Opportunities available for higher pay than at present. ■ Heads to be appraised also by governing body. ■ £1 billion announced to pay for the start of the new system.	Elements of managerialist ideology clearly apparent in these proposals. Portfolio preparation is fraught with already-documented problems. Clearly there is going to be a certain amount of creativity in relation to how these policies are actually implemented at the ground level if this Green Paper becomes law in this form.
May 1999 Government announces proposals for 'Curriculum 2000', a slimmed-down version of the national curriculum	Follows from the *Qualifying for Success* consultation, discussed above. Curriculum 2000 to be implemented in September 2000 when finally agreed. Implements the broader A level structure set out above.	Widely criticized as too complex, with insufficient time for implementation. However, there was wide support for the measures which were in line with those proposed by DES (1988) but rejected by the Thatcher administration.

| March 1999 *Excellence in Cities* initiative announced | Targeted at Key Stages 3, 4 and 5. Planned to:

■ develop and expand the number of beacon and specialist schools
■ extend opportunities for gifted and talented children
■ launch a new network of learning centres
■ encourage setting by schools (i.e. a form of internal selectivism)
■ give a new emphasis to literacy and numeracy teaching
■ introduce a scheme of low-cost home computer lease for pupils and adults who face particular disadvantages
■ strengthen school leadership
■ turn around the weakest schools
■ modernize LEAs
■ tackle disruption in schools more effectively by ensuring every school has access to a Learning Support Unit
■ provide a 'learning mentor' for every young person who needs one, as a single point of contact to tackle barriers to pupils' learning
■ introduce new, smaller Education Action Zones to focus on low performance in small clusters of schools | Initiative broadly welcomed, with head teachers in particular responding enthusiastically to extra resources. The first annual report in 2001 on the scheme identifies considerable success. This is available from: http://www.standards.dfes.gov.uk/excellence/.

Details of beacon schools are available at: http://www.standards.dfes.gov.uk/ beaconschools/. |

continued

Table 1.1 *continued*

Key policy events	Selected key content	Commentary
March 1999 *Excellence in Cities* initiative announced (continued)	■ provide subsidised loans to teachers for the purchase of computers September 1999: Phase One covers secondary schools in 25 LEAs. September 2000: a further 22 areas join up, along with primary pilots in Phase One areas. September 2001: a further 10 areas joined. Programme covered more than a thousand schools – about a third of all secondary-age pupils in the country.	
November 2000 National College for School Leadership announced	Immediately took charge of leadership training for schools which had since the mid-1990s been dispersed in regions around the country.	Broadly welcomed by the profession, though the underlying philosophy of management education underpinning the college appears to continue to be a rather dated competence-based one. The college website is at: http://www.ncsl.org.uk.
September 2001 *Schools – Achieving Success* White Paper published	The government plans to: ■ amend legislation to enable many more students to take Key Stage 3, GCSE and advanced qualifications earlier in their school lives to allow them to broaden or deepen their studies, spend more time	These proposals are presented under the following broad headings: ■ modernizing education law ■ high minimum standards for all ■ deregulation and diversity

on vocational options, undertake voluntary activity or move on to advanced level study early

■ amend existing legislation to promote greater rigour in tackling poor behaviour, in parallel with policies to encourage children, their parents and their schools to contribute to improved behaviour while learning

■ introduce legislation that allows schools greater freedom to establish governance arrangements that suit them

■ where legislative constraints prevent chools from sharing resources and expertise, loosen them so that schools can more easily work together, for example sharing an excellent team of subject teachers

■ legislate to allow for all-age City Academies and for schools on the City Academy model in disadvantaged rural as well as urban areas

■ take powers to allow successful schools greater freedoms to innovate, for example greater flexibility within clearly defined limits on pay and conditions and the curriculum, if this would support them to raise standards

■ meeting individual talents and aspirations at 14–19
■ building for excellence
■ early years and childcare
■ deregulating teacher employment provisions
■ teachers' pay.

continued

Table 1.1 continued

Key policy events	Selected key content
September 2001 Schools – Achieving Success White Paper published (continued)	■ introduce a right of appeal to the Adjudicator where a successful school's proposals for expansion are rejected by the School Organisation Committee ■ legislate to enable excellent schools to support and partner weak or failing schools in new ways ■ legislate to require LEAs to advertise widely when a new school is required, and for decisions on these competitions to be taken by the Secretary of State ■ provide a reserve power for the Secretary of State to require an LEA to involve an external partner in turning round a failing school ■ in cases of school weakness or failure, allow for a governing body to be replaced by an Interim Executive Board as part of a turn-around solution ■ legislate to make sure that there is sufficient curricular flexibility at Key Stage 4 to implement our proposals for 14–19 education ■ remove any legislative barriers to collaboration between schools and between schools and FE colleges so that, for example, there may be greater sharing of teaching staff ■ take legislative powers to remove any structural barriers to the creation of the 14–19 phase, including in its organisation, funding and inspection

continued

- make sure that students have access to high quality advice and guidance at key points of choice in order that they are better placed to take charge of their own decisions. Legislate to secure this if necessary.

- legislate to assist new teachers, working in shortage subjects in both schools and Further Education, who enter and remain in employment in the state sector, to pay off their student loans over a set period of time

- take powers to enable certain groups of teachers, for example trainees and teachers qualified abroad, to be registered with the General Teaching Council as well as strengthening the GTC's powers more generally

- take powers to require school place allocation to be co-ordinated by LEAs and all areas to have Admissions Forums. Also clarify and simplify key aspects of admissions law and guidance.

- legislate to refine powers that tackle failure and under-performance in LEAs

- legislate to define separate budgets for schools and LEA central functions, and for a Schools Forum to exercise functions in relation to the schools budget

- take a reserve power to allow the Secretary of State, in exceptional circumstances, to direct a local authority to set a budget for expenditure on schools at a level determined by the Secretary of State, having regard to all the relevant circumstances

Table 1.1 *continued*

Key policy events	Selected key content
September 2001 *Schools – Achieving Success* White Paper published (continued)	■ simplify and consolidate the Secretary of State's grant-making powers ■ legislate to free school governors to run a wide range of family and community facilities and services, including childcare ■ amend legislation for Early Years Partnerships to reflect their responsibilities for childcare ■ take powers to make the status of nursery schools more like that of other schools, for example as regards their governance and funding and to consolidate the Foundation Stage ■ legislate to replace the current baseline assessment arrangements with a single national end of Foundation Stage Profile based on the Early Learning Goals ■ enable co-operative approaches with other schools and institutions in Further and Higher Education by removing the assumption that schools provide education only through employing teachers ■ increase flexibility for permitting innovative approaches by providing for the main staffing provisions to be in secondary legislation and guidance ■ deregulate to allow more responsibility for staffing decisions in schools to shift from

the governing body to the head, in line with the proposals of the Way Forward Group on governance

- take forward the Way Forward Group proposal that the head should take decisions to dismiss staff, with an appeal to a committee of governors
- take power to set by order any standards to be attained by teachers at certain stages of their careers, subject to consultation but not to the pay machinery. This would take threshold, AST (Advanced Skills Teacher) and Fast Track teacher standards out of the STRB (School Teachers' Review Body) machinery. Take power to put into force, again subject to consultation, any administrative arrangements or procedures necessary to give effect to provisions relating to statutory pay and conditions.
- clarify the existing 'fast-track' procedure of consulting the Chair of the STRB to bring into force minor or consequential pay and conditions provisions, without formal reference to the STRB
- update the 1986 Act provision empowering the Secretary of State to make teacher appraisal regulations so that there is an explicit power for schools to use appraisal data in pay decisions, as well as technical updating
- make sure that head teachers can assess teachers' performance for pay purposes within the overall budgetary framework set by the governing body
- correct the removal of point 0 from the teachers' pay spine in 1999.

retained grammar and secondary modern schools. Some areas had a three-tier system, with a middle school stage between the primary and secondary stages. There were 34,000 schools in the UK. At both primary and secondary levels there were four main categories of maintained (state) schools in England and Wales. These were governed and funded in distinct ways:

- County schools: funded wholly through the LEA. After the advent of local management of schools (LMS) in 1988 LEAs delegated spending power and other responsibilities to governing bodies but retained powers of oversight and funding for various services.
- Voluntary controlled schools: owned by charities, usually churches. The LEA, however, retained considerable power over the schools.
- Voluntary aided schools: also owned by charities, usually churches. More control over school policies lay with the governing bodies of these schools than was the case with voluntary controlled schools.
- Grant-maintained schools: free from LEA control and funded (in England) by central government through the Funding Agency for Schools (FAS), an agency of the Department of Education and Employment. There were around 450 grant-maintained (GM) primary schools (3 per cent) and 650 GM secondary schools (20 per cent) in England.

Additionally at secondary level only there were city technology colleges which were also free from LEA control. They were funded by the Department for Education and Employment but promoters owned or leased the premises and were responsible for their management. There were only fifteen CTCs in existence, considerably fewer than the Conservative government planned for.

Parents could send their children to private schools if they could pay the fees. The assisted places scheme was designed to allow low-income families to take advantage of this option. Around 35,000 assisted places were made available annually in England and Wales.

Provision for most children with special needs was made in mainstream primary and secondary schools and, where possible, this was the favoured option. There were, however, special schools and colleges available to cater for special needs where necessary.

Policy and policy-making 1979–97

Policy-making is often thought about in terms of it being either *rational* or *incremental* in nature. The rational model assumes that policy-makers become aware of a problem, consider alternative ways of solving it and then choose the best (Etzioni 1967, p. 385). The incrementalist model by contrast sees policy-makers as 'muddling through' (Lindblom 1959). Policies change in reaction to changing circumstances and they can appear (and be) unco-ordinated, even contradictory. At one level it appears that the incrementalist view most closely models education policy-making during the 1944–79 period when there was broad consensus between Labour and Conservatives over many aspects of social policy (the 'Butskellite settlement'). There was only a limited ideological 'drive' behind policy-making, so decisions were arrived at through negotiation and compromise. However, after 1979 there was a clear shift in policy and policy-making away from that settlement towards a new, more radical vision for education and to a more rationalistic, co-ordinated, goal-oriented approach to policy-making in general.

Even after 1979 the rational model did not exist in a pure form. Policy-making is always a political process; competing groups, interests and ideologies continued to fight over the shape of education policy. In this context there was a clear tension between those who wanted central control and those who were more concerned with deregulation. Since the New Right (see p. 104) was politically and ideologically dominant and enjoyed a strong parliamentary majority, and many of the interest groups formerly involved in the policy process (e.g. teachers and the LEAs) were progressively marginalized, the ground over which this battle was fought was defined almost completely by New Right thinking and essentially involved the different factions within the New Right.

Table 1.2 shows how the respective roles of the players in education policy formulation changed over the years, with the trend being towards dominance at the centre.

The more co-ordinated, rationalist, nature of education policy

Table 1.2 Changing roles in the structure of education 1944–2001

	1944–74	1974–88	1988–97	1997–2001
Education Department	Overseers (chair)	Limited assertiveness	Minister's instrument	One among several interested departments
Political party in power	Reserve power	Electorally opportunist	Dominant	Dominant
LEA	Active partners (managing director)	Squeezed	Marginalized	Need to prove worth
Teachers	Active partners (executive director)	Problems	Proletarianized	Need to prove worth
Parents	Who?	Constructed as 'natural experts' or moral guardians	Consumers	Consumers
Industry	Indifferent (full employment)	Concerned (increasing unemployment)	Consultants	Partners

Source: Adapted from Dale 1989, p. 115

during this period is most evident in the links between the 1980, 1986 and 1988 Education Acts. What linked them was the idea of bringing market forces to education policy, with parents in the role of consumers. The case study below explores this key aspect of Tory education policy of the period.

The situation in 2001

After four years of Labour government, 1997–2001, remarkably little had changed in terms of compulsory education, the period seeing a continuation of much that the Conservatives had put in place. Ball (1999) notes that the basic organizing principles of Conservative policy remained in place:

- choice and competition: the commodification and consumerization of education
- autonomy and performativity: the managerialization and commercialization of education
- centralization and prescription: the imposition of centrally determined assessments, schemes of work and classroom methods.

The policy of encouraging schools to develop specialisms, linked to the theme of choice and competition, led to a trebling in the number of 'specialist' schools in that period, and this policy continued into Labour's second term (from 2001). The Conservatives' focus on the basics was retained too, with national strategies on literacy and numeracy in primary schools adopting what was, for their critics, a centralist and traditionalist approach to teaching and learning at that level.

One main difference was that the level of spending increased: the share of Gross Domestic Product (GDP) devoted to education overall increased from 4.6 per cent to 5 per cent, with total education spending increasing from just over £37 billion to nearly £50 billion between 1997 and 2001. Another was the special focus on disadvantaged schools: Labour's *Excellence in Cities* programme gave additional support to those schools which faced special issues associated with social and economic disadvantage in the areas from which they drew pupils. A third difference was a concern to update schools and to take full advantage of new technologies in education as was happening extremely rapidly in the economy as a whole. The government realized, however, that while investment in technological infrastructure, particularly through the National Grid for Learning (a government-funded resource aiming to make schools into a networked learning community through the internet), could be implemented relatively easily, the patchy levels of knowledge about and confidence with information and communication technology (ICT) among the teaching profession meant that getting it used well in schools was a more difficult task.

Case study: extending parental choice

Why extend parental choice?

Three key ideas underlay this aspect of Conservative policy:

- Teachers, local authority officers and others were running the education service in their own interests, not those of children and parents (summed up in the phrase 'producer capture').
- Schools had ceased to look outwards to their communities and had become insular.
- The combination of these factors had led to a complacent attitude in the education service, where low standards were accepted and motivation to improve was lacking.

Extending the rigours of the marketplace to the education service, it was thought, would force the service to look outwards to its market – parents. Schools would learn to offer what parents wanted or would go under, with good schools driving out the bad through the power of their success in the new education marketplace. The best schools would become dynamic, distinctive and beacons of excellence. The worst would simply close as parents took their children elsewhere.

How was it done?

- Empowering governing bodies. The powers, duties and responsibilities of governing bodies were expanded under the Education

Acts of 1980, 1985 and 1986. Simultaneously parents gained more seats on governing bodies. Interesting proposals very similar to these had been set out in the Taylor Report (1977), led by the Labour leader of Blackburn City Council reporting to a Labour government.

- Opening school doors to parents. Parents were given the right to select the school their children would attend, and schools were obliged to admit pupils up to a pre-defined number: this was called 'open enrolment'. Whether a child lived in the school's catchment area was now less important. Schools could reject children only on the grounds that they did not meet the entrance criteria or that the school was full.
- Making information available to parents. Schools now had to make public their aims, procedures, selection criteria, examination and test results, levels of truancy, etc. Parents had the right to see records about their children and receive a written report. School governors' reports also had to be published and a meeting held with parents at least once a year. Parents would now be able to make an informed choice.
- Imposing rigorous school inspection. Regular reports by independent inspectors were also partly intended to inform parents about the strengths and weaknesses of local schools and therefore to act as a basis for choice. Open meetings allowed parents to discuss their findings. Parents were sent a summary of the report and the full report was freely available (e.g. in local libraries).
- Extending parental right of appeal. Independent assessors on panels were appointed to hear appeals from parents unsuccessful in getting the school they wanted for their child.
- Creating different types of school. Setting up new forms of school such as grant-maintained schools and city technology colleges was designed partly to increase diversity and so give parents a greater range of choice.
- Rewarding success. The way schools were funded also changed. Most of the money schools received was now calculated on the basis of how many pupils they could attract. Successful, popular schools would thrive, unsuccessful ones would go into a cycle of decline and eventually close.
- Giving parents the right to vote. Parents were given the right to

vote for their child's school to opt out or not, i.e. to become grant-maintained or to stay under local authority control.

Did it work? The good news

The parents and school choice interaction (PASCI) project (Woods 1992; Woods et al. 1996) and the study by Gewirtz et al. (1995) found some evidence of success in these policies. Schools were now more likely to market themselves as 'a caring institution' or 'an academic institution', seeing this as providing what parents wanted. In other ways too the schools were catering for perceived parental demand, for example in seeking to provide extracurricular activities for children, being more aware of the need to protect children's belongings and taking action more quickly when pupils were disruptive or likely to disturb the education of others. The aim of rewarding excellent schools and highlighting those which need improvement also appeared to have met some success according to data from McPherson and Raab (1988a). Their study of parental choice in first-year admission to ten schools in Dundee and ten in Edinburgh found that:

- There has been a large outflow from secondary schools serving the least popular housing schemes into adjacent, often previously selective, schools; 70 per cent of placement requests were made by parents wishing to avoid the local catchment school.
- Substantial inequalities were developing among secondary schools which formerly had had equal status: magnet and sink schools were developing. The theory was that this would lead the 'sink' schools to improve their practices, to be taken over by a more effective 'task force' of managers and teachers or to close completely.

Did it work? The bad news

There are a number of problems with the ideas underpinning this strand of Conservative education policy. First is the very notion of education as a marketplace. Choosing a school, or deciding to take a child to another one, is unlike buying a new car, for example, in a number of important ways. Buying a car is not compulsory, and if something is wrong you can require the supplier to put right any defects. Your actions as purchaser do not affect the nature of the car.

Cars come in a wide range of styles and prices and you can shop around very effectively. The car itself has no say in the purchase arrangements. For these and other reasons the education system is at best a 'quasi-market'. Moreover there is a problem in trying to change the parent–school relationship into a market one: instead of a relationship of partnership and co-operation in which parents have a say in the education of their child, it becomes almost a conflictual one. Power et al.'s (1996) study of grant-maintained schools found that parents were marginalized and devalued by these supposedly market-driven schools. Deem (1996a) found that the attempt to empower governors had been neutralized by the increased power of state control over the national curriculum, assessment, funding and teachers' conditions.

However, critics of the Conservatives' parental choice policy have concentrated most on its detrimental effects on equality of opportunity, and the continuing importance of social disadvantage in conditioning educational achievement. Many commentators see such policies as developing an educational underclass, largely concentrated in the inner cities, who are unable to exercise a choice. They point to a number of reasons why this happens.

- In an effort to achieve high standards and so become more attractive to parents, schools become choosier too. During the 1990s they were allowed to select more children by ability; these procedures will disadvantage the already disadvantaged in much the same way as the grammar/secondary-modern system did. The PASCI project found clear evidence of this happening. Gewirtz et al. (1995) found that schools were using subtle methods to select parents and pupils, for example making application forms difficult to complete, setting early deadlines and making parents sign contracts of co-operation. All these meant that the more motivated, knowledgeable and literate parents were more likely to be successful.
- For the same reason schools will move quickly to exclude difficult pupils. The number of exclusions from school increased markedly in the 1990s as schools attempted to protect their reputations for discipline and good order locally. Disadvantaged children in particular will suffer from this.

- These policies reward success rather than offering support for disadvantaged schools. Schools situated in areas where parents do not want to send their children will suffer financially. A 1993 OFSTED (see Glossary) report found standards 'inadequate' and 'disturbing' in schools, colleges and other educational centres in a variety of city areas visited where there were 'pockets of severe disadvantage'.

- The market-driven emphasis on testing and streaming results in children being labelled at an early age, reinforcing teachers' expectations based on stereotypes about ethnicity and social class.

- Disadvantaged parents cannot exercise choice easily: lack of resources means they have to send their child to the local school. Some children from minority ethnic groups will not be able to attend schools with entry criteria related to religion.

- Parents who understand and know how to use educational information may be empowered by these policies. Others are not. The possession of cultural capital (see Glossary) becomes very important.

Conclusion: policy outcomes are highly variable

Most studies agree that large generalizations about the outcomes of policy such as that on parental choice are impossible. Local conditions have very important effects on whether a policy 'works' or not and can often result in unintended consequences. In some GM schools parental involvement has increased, in others it has diminished. In some areas LEA schools are highly attractive to parents, in others the GM schools are more attractive (Power et al. 1996). In some areas there is a highly active quasi-market, in others there is not (Woods et al. 1996). Conservative policies have increased equality of educational opportunity in some aspects of the educational service and reduced it in others (Arnot et al. 1996). Chapters 3 and 4 will show how this local reception of policy, its (re)interpretation and subsequent implementation are extremely important in (often) changing policy as it moves through its 'career'.

Key points

- There has been a shift away from the Butskellite settlement on education achieved after 1945 to a set of policies influenced by New Right ideology and largely excluding input from interest groups such as teachers and LEAs. This ideological position is found in the final years of Labour administration in the 1970s as well as in Conservative government policies in the 1980s, 1990s and 2000s. Their critics argue that the Labour governments of the late 1990s and early 2000s retain too much of the New Right legacy in the New Right/Social Democratic mix that characterizes New Labour.

- As the above point indicates, political ideology rather than negotiated settlement became increasingly important in education policy-making as well as in other areas of policy during the 1980s and 1990s.

- Partly as a result of this, policy-making achieved greater coherence and consistency in recent decades, though internal contradictions in education policies and 'muddling through' also continued to characterize the 1980s and 1990s.

- One key aspect of education policy, the introduction of market forces to the education system through the enhancement of parental choice, has had a number of unintended outcomes.

- Legislation has become more all-encompassing in character over the years and the rate of policy development and change has become increasingly frenetic.

- But outcomes are complex and tend to be shaped by ground-level characteristics as well as by the policy itself.

Guide to further reading

For a good summary of reports, legislation and the education system as a whole see:

Mackinnon, D. and Statham, J. (1999) *Education in the UK: Facts and figures*, London: Hodder and Stoughton, in association with the Open University (3rd edition).

---

continued

For a collection of important documents see:
Maclure, S. (ed.) (1986) *Educational Documents, England and Wales, 1816 to the Present Day*, London: Methuen, 5th edition.

For an overview of the 1988 Education Act see:
Maclure, S. (1989) *Education Re-formed: A Guide to the Education Reform Act*, London: Hodder and Stoughton, 2nd edition.

For a summary of the latest legislation see:
Croner (no single date) *The Teacher's Legal Guide*, Kingston-upon-Thames: Croner.
Taylor, G., Saunders, J. B. and Liell, P. (annually) *The Law of Education*, London: Butterworth.

For current information about education in the UK and Europe see:
Government Statistical Office (annually) *Social Trends*, London: HMSO.
Organisation for Economic Co-operation and Development (annually) *Education at a Glance*, Paris: OECD.

For a series of interesting studies on the impact of policies in schools see:
Pole, C. and Chawla-Duggan, R. (eds) (1996) *Reshaping Education in the 1990's: Perspectives on Primary Schooling*, London: Falmer Press.
Pole, C. and Chawla-Duggan, R. (eds) (1996) *Reshaping Education in the 1990's: Perspectives on Secondary Schooling*, London: Falmer Press.

For a discussion of the contradictions within the 1988 Education Act see:
Coulby, D. and Bash, L. (1991) *Contradiction and Conflict: The 1988 Education Act in Action*, London: Cassell.

For an insight see:
Lawton, Denis (1994) *The Tory Mind on Education, 1979–94*, London: Falmer Press.
Lawson distinguishes between three strands of Tory thinking on education: the privatizers, the minimalists and the pluralists. Using some interesting primary material Lawton sets out the views of politicians who represent each of these, often in their own words. Providing a useful analytical framework, Lawton traces the development of Tory education

policy over the period he covers and then discusses the future in a way which provokes the reader into considering the options carefully. Thus, while giving a readable account of policies, the book contextualizes and structures them in a way which is extremely valuable.

Useful addresses
OFSTED Publications Centres

Free Publications
OFSTED Publications Centre
Orders: 07002 637833
Fax: 07002 693274
E-mail: freepublications@ofsted.gov.uk

Priced Publications
The Stationery Office – TSO (formerly HMSO)
Offices throughout the country. Look in the phone book for your local branch.
Orders: 0870 600 5522
Fax: 0870 600 5533
Internet: http://www.official-documents.co.uk

Useful websites

http://www.standards.dfes.gov.uk/
The education standards website gives full details of many initiatives, particularly those undertaken between 1997 and 2002

http://www.legislation.hmso.gov.uk/acts.htm
Acts of the UK Parliament: full text of all public and local Acts going back to 1988 and 1991, respectively

http://www.labour.org.uk/
This is the Labour Party website

http://www.niss.ac.uk/
The NISS information gateway, for schools, FE and HE funding bodies, libraries, etc. National Information Services and Systems is an online information service for the UK education sector

http://www.sosig.ac.uk/
SOSIG (pronounced 'sausage') is the gateway to a number of extremely useful social science resources
http://www.parliament.the-stationery-office.co.uk/
The page for details on TSO (formerly HMSO) publications

http://www.parliament.uk/hophome.htm
The Parliament page

http://www.ofsted.gov.uk
The home page of the Office for Standards in Education. OFSTED reports on specific schools can be downloaded from here

http://www.ukonline.gov.uk/
The website from which a large range of information about government activities can be accessed; there is a very useful search engine here which will locate documents and information on a huge range of issues

http://www.dfes.gov.uk/
The website of the Department for Education and Skills

http://www.tes.co.uk/
The *Times Educational Supplement*'s website for the latest news and commentary on compulsory (and some post-compulsory) education

http://education.guardian.co.uk//
The home page of the *Guardian* newspaper's education website

Chapter 2
Policies and structures
Post-compulsory education

OUTLINE
This chapter sets out the background to the current post-compulsory education system in the UK, focusing on higher and further education and adult education, as well as, to some extent, youth training. It gives a summary of some policy landmarks of the eighteen years of Conservative government, 1979–97, as well as the first term of Labour office following that, 1997–2002. It then explores a case study of post-compulsory policy during that period. Finally the key points of the chapter are highlighted. It is important to note that although this chapter and Chapter 1 concentrate on legislative and other formal policy events, subsequent chapters go on to show that policy should be conceived in broader terms than simply the formal actions of government and other official agencies.

Background to the current system

In the late seventeenth century there were only two universities in England (Oxford and Cambridge), and four in Scotland (Edinburgh, Glasgow, St Andrews and Aberdeen). Even by the late eighteenth century there were only fourteen universities in total in the UK, although by now there were twenty thousand students (Scott 1995). The 'redbrick' universities, such as Leeds and Manchester, were founded in the latter part of the nineteenth century. Likewise the expansion of adult education towards the current situation in Britain began only in the nineteenth century. In 1821 the first technical ('mechanics') institute was set up (in Edinburgh). By 1850 there were 610 of these institutions, the precursors of today's further education colleges, around the country. Many would later become museums, libraries or polytechnics as well as technical or further education colleges. They were often funded by private donations and their aim was to improve the skills and knowledge of working people, particularly working men.

It is clear that the development of post-compulsory education was linked to the rise of industrial capitalism in the UK; the earlier forms of economic systems did not require large numbers of people with an advanced education, although from the seventeenth century onwards there had been a movement to educate adults so that they could read the Bible, especially amongst Quakers and Methodists. Indeed, a suspicion of the possible consequences of educating large numbers of the working class continued to pervade discussions about the expansion of education throughout the nineteenth century. These fears were diminished somewhat by the continuing religious function of education of adults and children: 'education for salvation' (Kelly 1983).

Other institutions, such as London Working Men's College and Leicester College (now the extra-mural teaching centre for Leicester University), were set up during the nineteenth century with a liberal arts focus, sometimes as a reaction to the vocationalism of the mechanics' institutes. From the 1870s university extra-mural work became increasingly important in non-vocational adult education. (Extra-mural, literally 'beyond the walls', means education for the community outside the university.) Subjects such as Greek, Latin, history, logic, literature and modern languages were taught.

The Workers' Education Association (WEA) was created in 1903, supported by the co-operative movement, trade unions and universities. The work of the WEA was rooted in the liberal humane philosophy of the universities. From 1924 the WEA gained funding from central government and began to split from the universities.

In 1919 the University Grants Committee was established. Its task was to distribute Treasury funds to the universities, at first on a small scale. It effectively acted as a buffer between the government and universities, ensuring that their work was free of political interference while allowing them the freedom which would enable them to become the important force they were to become later in the century. By 1938, on the eve of the Second World War, 2 per cent of 18 year olds attended university, but the figure for *female* 18 year olds was only 0.5 per cent (Blackburn and Jarman 1993).

Postwar expansion

The period after the war saw a large expansion in post-compulsory education. Section 41 of the 1944 Education Act (the Butler Act) made it:

> the *duty* of every local education authority to secure the provision for their area of adequate facilities for further education, that is to say, (i) Full-time and part-time education for persons over compulsory school age; and (ii) *Leisure time occupation* in such organised *cultural training and recreative activities* as are suited to their requirements, for any persons over compulsory school age *who are able and willing to profit* by the facilities provided for that purpose.
>
> (Emphasis mine)

Section 42 required local education authorities to co-operate with other providers, and section 53 emphasized the need for 'adequate facilities for recreation and social and physical training to be established in co-operation with voluntary agencies'.

The 1945 Percy Report considered the need for and provision of higher technological education in England and Wales. Its recommendations included the expansion of science teaching in universities and the creation of colleges of advanced technology. It also recommended that organizations should be established to co-ordinate the work of the various institutions involved in higher technological education at local and national levels. There was, simultaneously, a concern for the expansion of education as a recreation. The 1944 Education Act set up adult education centres offering a wide range of provision. The number of adult students in evening institutes rose from three hundred thousand in 1947 to more than a million in 1967, many studying on non-vocational courses. By that time the university system was undergoing rapid change. The newer civic universities, such as Newcastle and Leicester, were founded after the Second World War, often through the 'promotion' of an existing college.

Table 2.1 *Post-compulsory policy: some landmarks since 1979*

Key policy events	Selected key content	Commentary
1981 Expenditure White Paper announced cuts in university sector imposed by University Grants Committee	The University Grants Committee was faced with the having to apportion a cut of around 15% in total across the university sector. The intake of students was cut.	The unintended effect was to push students across the binary divide into the polytechnics where the government had not been able to control the number of places offered. Polytechnic student numbers expanded as a result.
1981 White Paper: *A New Training Initiative*	Youth Training Scheme (YTS) replaced a variety of schemes for 16–17 year olds who would otherwise probably have been unemployed. Began as a one-year scheme, subsequently (1986) increased to two.	Successful in terms of number of trainees (376,000 by 1988 but declining thereafter) and beset by problems (see p. 90).
1985 Jarratt Report	Charged with reviewing and making recommendations about university management, it recommended a raft of measures designed to make universities more effective and efficient through clearer management structures and styles.	Widely seen as the start of the application of managerialism (Pollitt 1990 and 1993 – see below) to the university sector. Though it had little measurable effect at the time, it marked a change in attitudes and discourse about university management.

1985 Green Paper *The Development of Higher Education into the 1990s*	Accepted the polytechnics and universities funding bodies' redefinition of the Robbins principle to become 'courses of higher education should be available to all those who can benefit from them and who wish to do so' with the proviso that the benefit justifies the cost.	A move towards accepting expansion of the higher education system after the cuts of the early 1980s, but within clearly limited spending. The government was attempting here to tackle the dilemma of catering for the demand for higher education while containing escalating costs now that it was moving beyond a small 'elite' system. This issue proved to be an ongoing one into the 1990s and would be tackled by the 1997 Dearing Report (see p. 63).
1986 National Council for Vocational Qualifications (NCVQ) set up after the White Paper *Working Together: Education and Training* is published	NCVQ established after the 1986 MSC/DES Review of Vocational Qualifications. Its remit was: ■ the establishment of a National Vocational Qualification framework which is comprehensible and comprehensive, and facilitates access, progression and continued learning ■ the improvement of vocational qualifications themselves, based on standards of competence required in employment.	Set up a system of vocational qualifications ranging from Level 1 (basic craft) to Level 5 (equivalent to postgraduate professional vocational qualifications) which were approved but not directly offered by the NCVQ. Based on the demonstrated achievement of vocational competence, identified in a series of explicit learning outcomes. Subsequently expanded to cover most vocational qualifications with a total of over a million National Vocational Qualifications awarded by 1995 (Robinson 1996, p. 5). However, this proved to be a highly contentious approach to training which, if extended to higher education, will be even more so.

continued

Table 2.1 continued

Key policy events	Selected key content	Commentary
1987 White Paper *Higher Education: Meeting the Challenge*	The priority throughout was to reform the HE system to meet the economic needs of the country. 'Meeting the needs of the economy is not the sole purpose of higher education nor can higher education alone achieve what is needed. But this aim, with its implications for the scale and quality of higher education, must be vigorously pursued . . . The Government and its central funding agencies will do all they can to encourage and reward approaches by higher education institutions which bring them closer to the world of business.'	This reviewed the whole spectrum of higher education, the fullest review since the 1963 Robbins Report and until the 1997 Dearing Report. Many of its proposals were translated into legislation through the 1988 Education Act.
1987 DES/Welsh Office publishes *Managing Colleges Efficiently*	Recommends: ■ the use of 'efficiency indicators': clear quantitative measures of inputs and outcomes ■ the use of 'efficiency targets' to be able to measure achievement by making objectives clear ■ improvements to information systems and statistics	A further move towards managerialist ethos, this time in the further education sector. This built on the work of the Audit Commission *Obtaining Better Value From Colleges* which indicated that efficiency savings could be made but was not tasked to indicate how this could be done. This paper, however, gives clear proposals which lay the ground for legislation.

1987 DES/Welsh Office publishes *Managing Colleges Efficiently* (continued)

- that managers should have the power to control and allocate resources with freedom from detailed external control (for example by the LEA).

This paralleled TVEI not just organizationally but in terms of its aims. The idea was to vocationalize higher education, integrating 'enterprise' into degree schemes more generally so that every student has experience of the economy and becomes 'a person who has belief in his [*sic*] own destiny, welcomes change and is not frightened of the unknown, sets out to influence events, has powers of persuasion, is of good health, robust, with energy and willing to work beyond that which is specified, is competitive, is moderated by concern for others and is rigorous in self-evaluation' (MSC Press Release, 1987).

1987 Announcement of the Enterprise in Higher Education initiative

Like TVEI (see p. 7) set up under the Manpower Services Commission (now TEED) this aimed to increase the supply of university graduates 'with enterprise'. A series of five-year schemes ran in universities and polytechnics with considerable amounts of pump-priming money attached to them. These began to wind down in the mid-1990s.

continued

Table 2.1 continued

Key policy events	Selected key content	Commentary
1988 Education Act	■ Polytechnics freed from LEA control. ■ Universities Funding Council and Polytechnic and Colleges Funding Councils established (UGC (Universities' Grant Committee) abolished in 1989 and these two councils merged in 1992). ■ Tenure can no longer be granted to protect academics' jobs.	This Act laid the foundations for the 1992 Act by moving the polytechnics' status towards that of the universities. Continued the managerialist thrust within universities by undermining one of the safeguards to academic freedom.
1988 White Paper: *Employment for the 1990s*	Set out the nature and functions of the new Training and Enterprise Councils (TECs; Local Enterprise Councils, LECs, in Scotland), charged to meet community's needs and government objectives with regard to vocational education and training.	TECs set up over a 3-year period from 1989. There were 76 TECs in England and Wales and 22 LECs in Scotland. They each had between £15 million and £55 million to devote to training in their area under the direction of the Training, Enterprise and Education Directorate (TEED) nationally. The TECs were disbanded in 2001, their functions being taken over by Small Business Service (SBS) areas, Learning and Skills Councils and Welsh Economic Regions. In Scotland, however, the LECs continue their work. No similar bodies exist in Northern Ireland.

1989 CBI paper *Towards a Skills Revolution*	The Confederation of British Industry advocated the introduction of Training Credits for 16–18 year olds.	A training credit is an individual entitlement to train to approved standards for 16 and 17 year olds who have left full-time education to join the labour market. Each credit displays a monetary value and can be used by a young person to obtain training with an employer or training provider. The aims of training credits are: ■ to expand and improve training by motivating more young people to train and to train to higher standards ■ to increase the quantity and quality of training provided for young people by employers ■ to establish an efficient market in training (Hall 1994, p. 194).
1990 Education (Student Loans) Act	Empowers Secretaries of State to make arrangements for higher education students to receive and repay loans towards their maintenance while studying.	An important piece of legislation which marked a shifting of the burden of the costs of the expanded higher education towards the 'consumer': students. Again this attempted to address the issue of how to pay for the enlarged system.

continued

Table 2.1 continued

Key policy events	Selected key content	Commentary
1990 RSA paper *More Means Different*	Stressed the need to widen access to higher education in a competitive international economic environment. Returns to the theme of the Higginson Report (see p. 10) about the inappropriateness of A levels in that context.	Often used as a reference point by those keen to promote the expansion of higher education.
1991 White Paper *Higher Education: A New Framework*	Reaffirmed the views set out in *Meeting the Challenge* and signalled the move to 'cost effective expansion': 'the general need to contain public spending, the pattern of relative costs in higher education, and the demands for capital investment, all mean that a continuing drive for greater efficiency will need to be secured' (DES 1991b, pp. 10–12).	Described by Martin Trow as 'a document of hard managerialism' (Trow 1994, p. 13), this concentrated on the 'human capital' functions of universities rather than their liberal ideals and stressed the need for strong management in the pursuit of effective and efficient provision.
	Many of the structural and other 'reforms' set out in the 1992 FHE Act are announced here. The aim is for 30% of age grade to attend university by end of century.	According to Pollitt (1990) 'Managerialism is a set of beliefs and practices, at the core of which burns the seldom tested assumption that better management will prove an effective solvent for a wide range of economic

1991 White Paper *Education and Training for the Twenty-first Century*

Set out the rationale and recommendations for the independence of college and changes to funding of adult education set out in the 1992 Act. Also set out the rationale for the further development of NVQs and training credits.

and social ills.' It stresses increased productivity through stringent control of the production process by managers who are given the power to manage. The three Es are paramount: economy, efficiency and effectiveness. Careful, measurable, target setting, quantification of inputs and outputs and of performance is stressed, as is rewarding increasing efficiency.

Underpinned by neo-liberal thinking, the two parts of the White Paper claim that 'the individual is at the heart' of the policies they set out. The 1992 Act which followed aimed to further establish a vigorously competitive further and higher education system. Training credits and Youth Credits would begin to take over from conventional Youth Training, with Modern Apprenticeship schemes being funded through them rather than directly from central government or its agencies.

continued

Table 2.1 *continued*

Key policy events	Selected key content	Commentary

1992 Further and Higher Education Act	■ Polytechnics permitted to change name to University.
	■ New funding bodies set up (Higher Education Funding Councils and Further Education Funding Council).
	■ Council for National Academic Awards abolished.
	■ Further Education becomes independent of LEAs.
	■ Funding of adult education tied to limited range of courses:
	  – vocational qualifications; GCSE or GCE A/AS levels
	  – access courses preparing students for entry to a course of higher education
	  – courses which prepare students for the previous three categories
	  – basic literacy in English
	  – teaching English to students where English is not the language spoken at home
	  – basic principles of mathematics; independent living and communication skills (Hall 1994, p. 87).
		The most important single Act to affect further and higher education during the Conservative administrations. In this sense it is the equivalent of the 1988 Education Reform Act for schools. It abolished the binary divide between polytechnics and universities, signalling a reduction in funding for the latter as the playing field is levelled downwards.
		
		The incorporation of further education colleges would herald a period during which many of them would suffer great financial hardships and a fundamental restructuring of their staffing as many staff are encouraged to leave and are replaced by part-time or short-term contract staff.
		
		Adult education was forced to 'vocationalize' its provision so as to continue to receive funding after this Act. Many adult students object to this and to the fact that awards (and examinations and other forms of assessment) now become attached to what were simply courses enjoyed for their own sake.

November 1993 'Autumn Statement' on funding	■ Government announces cut of 45% in student fees to universities. ■ Universities to be penalized for under- or over-recruiting target numbers of students, making it financially unattractive to recruit more students. ■ The planned number of places to be offered in 1994 was reduced by 10,000. ■ Funding council grants and student grants also to be cut (Richards 1993; CVCP 1993).	The government's response to the escalating costs of the free market in higher education which it had established was now to put on the brakes through this funding strategy. It now planned for stasis in student numbers for three years after a period of very rapid expansion in the early 1990s.
1994 White Paper *Competitiveness*	■ Proposed 'accelerated modern apprenticeships' for 18 and 19 year olds with A levels or GNVQs. These will lead to qualifications at NVQ Level 3. ■ Proposal to spend £300 million on this expansion between 1997 and 1998.	By 1997 the government had introduced the Modern Apprenticeship scheme for the work-based training in skills needed by technicians and supervisory staff. The apprentice, the employer and the TEC sign an 'apprenticeship pledge' describing the training to be provided and committing all parties to it. The training is based on the competence model. Around 90% of expenditure on employment training for young people was spent on Modern Apprenticeships, with Youth Training accounting for the rest by 1997.

continued

Table 2.1 *continued*

Key policy events	Selected key content	Commentary
1996 Dearing Report on Qualifications for 16 to 19 Year Olds (second Dearing Report – see p. 14 for first and Chapter 5 for third)	This report concluded that: ■ a number of education and training initiatives have had modest success. In particular Youth Training and National Records of Achievement need to be re-structured and re-launched. ■ the framework for all qualifications for 16–19 year olds needs to be simplified into a system of National Levels. All certificates issued by awarding bodies should show which of four National Levels the award is at (advanced; intermediate; foundation; entry). ■ quality assurance structures and procedures with this national framework should be simplified and rationalized. SCAA and NCVQ should be merged for example. (This was incorporated into the 1997 Education Act.) ■ a distinctive diploma at advanced level should be introduced which would give access to breadth of study at this level (see the	A key theme of this report is the sheer complexity of education and training at this level, the unnecessary multiplication of agencies, names, awards, awarding and assessing bodies and the proliferation of jargon. This makes the system very difficult to understand for students, teachers and potential employers and undermines its effectiveness. From a policy sociology point of view this is the almost inevitable result of the micropolitics of education policy-making and its implementation. Agencies vie with one another, impose their own agendas and interpretations on policy initiatives and seek to maximize their own gains. The result is a highly complex set of structures and processes. The report recommends that government should attempt to impose order on this chaos. The National Council for Vocational Qualifications (NCVQ) attempted to do this for vocational qualifications in particular, imposing a five-level structure on qualifications from a

	commentary on the Higginson Report, p. 10). In addition to two A levels or a full GNVQ or NVQ, students would have complementary 'breadth' studies at AS level. ■ the term GNVQ should be replaced by 'applied A level' and some changes should be made to GNVQs to improve rates of completion. ■ NVQs should be further developed to incorporate 'key skills' (IT, communication and number) and more underpinning knowledge and understanding rather than just ability to perform tasks.	variety of awarding bodies. It has, however, only been partly successful in its attempt to simplify vocational qualifications (Robinson 1996). Entropy appears to be endemic in the British education system.
1996 Education (Student Loans) Act	Allowed students to borrow from banks on the same terms as from the Student Loans Company. Banks bid to provide loans through competitive tendering process.	A move toward 'privatizing' student loans after criticism of the Student Loans Company and its handling (and recovery) of the loans. By now it was becoming clear that the burden of higher education was going to be shouldered by students and that HE was increasingly seen as a 'positional' rather than a 'public' good: i.e. one which primarily benefits the individual rather than society as a whole and therefore should be paid for by the individual.

continued

Table 2.1 *continued*

Key policy events	Selected key content	Commentary
1997 Election of Labour government. Kennedy Report *Learning Works*	Published by the Further Education Funding Council, the report of the committee chaired by Helena Kennedy QC proposed that: ■ there should be a greater level of participation in further education ■ further education should attract more funding and students should be properly provided for ■ ambitious targets should be set, with NVQ Level 3 becoming the norm ■ the government should take an important strategic as well as funding role in this, partly by creating coherent systems of information and a common credit system.	The report argued strongly that learning, particularly in further education, is the key to economic prosperity and social cohesion. In this it probably overestimated the power of education to compensate for social and economic circumstances (see pp. 164–7 for more on this). The report created concern in higher education circles that funding would be channelled away from higher and towards further education, which was in a period of crisis at this time. Though there was some evidence that the government did shift the emphasis of funding in this way, this was not a result of the report. Although the government is committed to an additional half million students, mostly to FE, and has found an extra £110 million for FE and £140 million for HE since it came to office, there are still doubts about the commitment to fund the vision in the Kennedy Report. The Government's response to the report is at: http://www.lifelonglearning. co.uk/kennedy/index.htm.

1997 Dearing Report	Recommended:	The new Labour government was quick to implement funding changes which placed more of the burden on students. These changes have since been heavily criticized for their negative effects on the widening participation strategy.
	■ the expansion of the higher education system with more of the national income spent on it	Government announced the introduction of tuition fees for students of £1,000 per year, to be introduced from 1998. These to be means-tested and repaid when the individual was in employment. The maintenance grant to be phased out.
	■ students should bear part of the cost of their higher education	
	■ there should be greater selectivity in funding for research	Announcement of 500,000 new places in higher education by the end of the century by the Prime Minister, but universities subsequently had difficulty filling places.
	■ universities should collaborate, not compete	
	■ a new qualifications framework to be established	The government's full response to the report, published in 1998, is available at: http://www.lifelonglearning.co.uk/dearing/index.htm. For further discussion see *Times Higher Education Supplement*, 27 February 1998, pp. 1, 7, 10, 11, 18.
	■ greater provision for lifelong learning	
	■ better teaching and more ICT to be introduced into universities	
	■ objectives and outcomes of higher education to be made clearer to students, employers and others.	For a discussion of the progress towards the goals set out in the Dearing Report since its publication, see *Times Higher Education Supplement*, 24 July 1998, pp. 4 and 5.

continued

Table 2.1 *continued*

Key policy events	Selected key content	Commentary
September 1997 Announcement of an additional £165 million for higher education to make good in part the funding gap	This was aimed at fulfilling the government's promise to make good the funding gap in higher education: resources had been declining relative to student numbers for some years and it seemed that the new arrangements for funding higher education (student fees plus the gradual abolition of student grants) would not benefit higher education financially.	Universities continued to threaten to introduce 'top-up' fees, arguing that they were not seeing enough of the money which resulted from government measures, and that this announcement of £165 million would be insignificant given the number of institutions and students in the system by the late 1990s.
November 1997 Government announces additional funding of £83 million for further education	The financial crisis hitting further education since incorporation in 1992 was severe (see p. 58). This announcement went some way to addressing this issue.	The Further Education Funding Council had made it clear that the FE sector was in a serious state, with a dramatically increasing number of colleges in financial trouble. The unit of resource (funding per student) had declined by around a third since incorporation. By 1997 the sector had changed in important, and often negative, ways.
February 1998 *The Learning Age* Green Paper on lifelong learning	Government sets out its vision of 'a learning society in which everyone, from whatever background, routinely	

expects to learn and upgrade their skills throughout life'.

Key principles of the Green Paper are:

■ 500,000 extra people in FE/HE by 2002

■ creation and launch of the University for Industry (Ufl) by late 1999 (see http://www.ufiltd.co.uk)

■ individual learning accounts to be set up to encourage people to save to learn

■ more young people to continue to study beyond age 16 with government help

■ financial support for basic literacy and numeracy skills amongst adults to be doubled. Half a million people to be involved by 2002

■ participation to be widened in further, higher, adult and community education

■ new Training Standards Council to be set up to raise standards in post-compulsory teaching and learning, inspection in further and adult education to be instituted

■ targets for the nation's skills and qualifications to be published

Key criticisms of the Green Paper are:

■ Cost implications of proposals have limited what is envisaged (the paper has been 'written by the Treasury' according to Phil Willis, Lib Dem spokesman.)

■ The paper envisages turning universities into FE colleges, concerned with lower-level skills and knowledge.

For further discussion see *Times Higher Education Supplement*, 27 February 1998, pp. 1, 7, 10, 11, 18.

The individual learning accounts scheme, set up in 2000 following this Green Paper, had to be abolished by late 2001 because it gave rise to a considerable amount of fraudulent acitivity and loss of public money.

continued

Table 2.1 *continued*

Key policy events	Selected key content	Commentary
February 1998 *The Learning Age* Green Paper on lifelong learning. (continued)	■ business, employees and trade unions involved in developing and supporting workplace skills ■ simplify the post-compulsory qualifications system and give equal value to both academic and vocational learning.	At the last minute this was demoted from the status of White Paper (well worked-out proposals prior to the publication of a Bill) to Green Paper. It was also several months late. The reason seems to have been government qualms about the potential costs. Learndirect evolves from the University for Industry initiative. Learndirect is designed to deliver learning to people at a place and pace to suit them, with considerable emphasis on information and communication technology helping this to happen. See http://www.learndirect.co.uk/.

Education (Student Loans) Act 1998	Transfers public sector student loans to the private sector, though under conditions set out by the government.	Follows severe criticism of the administration of student loans since they were instituted.
Teaching and Higher Education Act 1998	■ Sets up and defines the functions of the General Teaching Councils for England, for Wales and for Scotland. ■ Sets out the scheme for qualifications for head teachers. ■ Sets out new scheme for qualifications for teachers and induction arrangements for them. ■ Sets out new arrangements for financial support for HE students. ■ Sets out scheme for student fees at higher education institutions. ■ Introduces new legislation on time off work for study or training. ■ Sets out new powers for funding councils. ■ Legislates on the issue of the 'university' title, raised by the Dearing Report.	Interestingly the 'University for Industry' (see above) falls foul of the new regulations on the use of the 'university' title, being effectively part of the further education provision.

continued

Table 2.1 *continued*

Key policy events	Selected key content	Commentary
Budget March 1998	An extra £250 million announced for education, bringing the total to an extra £2.5 billion since Labour took office. More money announced for information technology skills training (most affecting further education) and for research and commercial development (£100 million and £50 million respectively). An additional £100 million announced for the New Deal for over 25 year old unemployed people. Some of this will involve further education training.	Despite worries that other measures in the budget concerning National Insurance contributions would prove expensive for education institutions, these measures were broadly welcomed. There appears to be congruence between these financial measures and educational policy, particularly in terms of lifelong learning.
July 1998 Announcement of the government's Comprehensive Spending Review (CSR) outcomes	£445 million extra for higher education over 1998–2000. University research to receive an increase of £1.4 billion over three years, some to come from the Wellcome Trust. Further education and sixth form colleges to receive an additional £225 million – an 8.2% cash increase on previous plans.	See *Times Higher Education Supplement*, 17 July 1998, for full account and discussion of the CSR as it applies to HE. The following week's edition (24 July) contains a commentary. Critical comment centres on the fact that the costs of these increases will fall largely on students via tuition fees.

November 1998 Announcement of expansion of FE and more funding for that sector	Government now plans to spend an extra £584 million on FE in 2000–1 but will expect an extra 200,000 students: this is an increase on earlier announcements of the outcome of the CSR (see above). Total to be invested in FE over 1999–2001 is now £908 million. Aim is to widen participation, improve standards of teaching and management, invest in ICT and support students with costs such as childcare.	The announcement failed to meet the hopes of colleges, but comes some way to meeting the difficult financial situation of many of them.
4 March 1999 The Higher Education Funding Council for England (HEFCE) earmarks £95 million out of next year's settlement to encourage universities to provide more places for poorer students	Change of funding mechanism designed to recognize the role of universities in broadening and deepening access, and the particular costs of this function.	This policy likely to benefit 'new' universities in particular. A welcome recognition of their particular mission and the costs this mission has for institutions.
July 1999 *Learning to Succeed: A New Framework for Post-16 Education* White Paper	It proposes: ■ setting up a Learning and Skill Council for England in 2001 with local Learning and Skills Councils too. Training and Enterprise Councils (TECs) to be replaced.	

continued

Table 2.1 *continued*

Key policy events	Selected key content	Commentary
July 1999 *Learning to Succeed: A New Framework for Post-16 Education* White Paper (continued)	■ new system of funding and planning post-16 education involving Regional Development Agencies (RDAs) ■ new inspection arrangements overseen by OFSTED ■ a 'Learning Gateway' for 16 and 17 year olds who need additional support ■ a new service of personal advisers to post-16s ■ close involvement of the University for Industry (UfI) with these developments ■ local businesses to be closely involved with these developments also ■ new Learning and Skills Councils to be closely involved in promoting Lifelong Learning. Full details are available at: www.lsc.gov.uk	

June 1999 Bett Report on pay and conditions in UK higher education.	Recommended the setting up of an independent pay review body, addressing the low pay of women in higher education and rectifying the decline in academic pay relative to other professions.	Very little response and no action was immediately evident from government on the basis of findings or recommendations. Prior to the 2001 election the government began to move on the pay review body issue.
15 February 2000 David Blunkett delivers Greenwich speech	Sets out ideas for the future direction of higher education. Globalization, ICT and the knowledge economy are key themes. The speech is available in full at: http://cms1.gre.ac.uk/dfee/#speech	
Mid-October 2000 DfEE publishes EUniversity report	Proposes setting up collaborative e-university to compete with foreign universities establishing a strong e-presence.	*Times Higher Education Supplement*, 6 October 2000, leads with story 'Elite Universities Log Off From EUniversity'. There is commentary on the policy in the next issue, 13 October. That headline indicates that there is suspicion about the viability of the scheme, especially among the more prestigious of the pre-1992 universities.

continued

Table 2.1 *continued*

Key policy events	Selected key content	Commentary
November 2000 HEFCE reports seven thousand full-time university places unfilled	Report by NUS *Equal Access or Elitist Entry?* identifies fall in 1999 of 7% in applications from males of skilled, semi-skilled or unskilled background compared to 1997. Applications from black males from African and Caribbean backgrounds fell by 11% and 9% respectively. The imposition of student fees and withdrawal of means-tested maintenance grants was blamed by the NUS. More details in the *Times Higher Education Supplement*, 17 November 2000, 'Rising Debt Hits Access Efforts', p. 1.	The paradox of government policy which, on the one hand, seeks to widen participation and support lifelong learning while, on the other, making students pay more, has these quite predictable outcomes.
2000 Scottish Parliament acts on Cubie proposals (the Independent Committee of Inquiry into Student Finance) that student payment of tuition fees for universities should be abolished	Scottish parliament (Holyrood) decides the following: ■ the abolition of tuition fees paid in advance from October 2001 ■ the introduction of a graduate endowment scheme – students have to pay back fees after graduating and getting a job that pays over a specified annual limit (though some classes of students to be exempt)	This decision places other countries within the UK in a difficult position. It is now clear to potential students that it is possible to have a good university system without the burden of tuition fees falling on them. A further problem is that the scheme will discourage Scottish students from studying outside Scotland.

| | | students in Scotland to be entitled to an income of which a proportion would be available in the form of a means-tested grant or bursary for those eligible | Some disappointment was expressed within Scotland that the Cubie proposals had not been implemented in full. Many saw them as being watered down in the Scottish parliament. |

■ students in Scotland to be entitled to an income of which a proportion would be available in the form of a means-tested grant or bursary for those eligible

■ low-income students would have the right to claim unemployment benefit during the summer holidays.

Some disappointment was expressed within Scotland that the Cubie proposals had not been implemented in full. Many saw them as being watered down in the Scottish parliament.

The Cubie inquiry website is at: http://www.studentfinance.org.uk/.

Late 2000 to early 2001 *The Excellence Challenge*

Government consults on proposals for widening the participation of young people in HE. HEFCE has a similar *consultation exercise* on funding widening participation.

Learning and Skills Act 2000

Sets up the Learning and Skills Council for England and a series of local councils. Replaces the TECs and the FEFC. The local learning and skills councils will have a £2.6 billion budget to fund the systems in 2002–3.

continued

Table 2.1 *continued*

Key policy events	Selected key content	Commentary
Learning and Skills Act 2000 (continued)	National body: ■ is responsible for the education and training of 16–19 year olds ■ assesses priorities and establishes plans ■ oversees work-based training – the successor to youth training – comes under a national formula and set of rules. These plans will determine the funds for work-based training. ■ oversees the work of the sixth-form and FE colleges. ■ school sixth-form funding also moves under skills council control (in April 2002) but does not change the management or legal status of school sixth-forms. Schools stay with local authorities. The budget (£1.2 billion in 2000–1) moves to the Learning and Skills Council, giving it important controlling power.	The White Paper *Learning to Succeed* talked of a Learning and Skills Council 'to drive forward improvements in standards and bring greater coherence and responsiveness' to post-16 education and training. The legislation has been interpreted as an extension of government control. Secretary of State for Education and Employment can direct the Council on a range of issues.

The Robbins Report and 1960s expansion

By 1963 there were still only twenty-four universities in the country, with 15 per cent of all students going to only two, Oxford and Cambridge. However, the 1963 Robbins Report on higher education, which had been appointed to review the provision of full-time higher education and make proposals for its development, recommended expansion to tap the 'pool of talent' which was not yet going into higher education, particularly from the working class. (Other excluded groups received less attention from the Robbins committee.) It proposed more than doubling full-time student numbers (to 560,000) by 1980, as well as setting up a body to oversee the granting of degrees in non-university institutions. (The Council for National Academic Awards (CNAA) was set up in 1964 to do this.)

The Open University was established in Milton Keynes in 1969, and a group of new universities was built in the 1960s. The new institutions became known as the 'Shakespearean universities' because of their names: York, Lancaster, Warwick, Sussex, Essex, Kent. Other institutions were promoted to university status at around the same time (e.g. Bath, Aston and Salford). Meanwhile, as a result of the 1966 White Paper *A Plan for Polytechnics*, which continued the expansionist philosophy of the Robbins Report, many colleges of advanced technology were being promoted to become degree-awarding polytechnics (twenty-nine in total by 1980). Unlike the chartered, and therefore independent, universities, they were under the control of their LEAs. The 1972 White Paper *Higher Education: A Framework for Expansion* promoted the continued expansion of higher education student places.

Non-vocational and leisure education

By 1970 vocational education was under the control of LEAs and colleges of commerce, art and technology. Non-vocational education was taken care of by LEAs, university extra-mural departments and the WEA, all with financial assistance from central government. Around half of adult education became oriented to 'leisure', with courses such as cooking, flower arranging, yoga, painting, arts and crafts and assorted hobbies. The year 1973 probably marks the high point of this phase of adult education; the Russell Committee's report proposed that non-vocational adult education should expand to give a comprehensive service to enable education to be continued throughout a person's lifetime. By then, however, the political climate was changing and few of the Russell Report's recommendations were implemented.

The situation in the mid-1990s

Higher education

In 1996 there were 176 higher education institutions in the UK, of which 115 were titled universities (which included the various constituent parts of the University of London and the University of Wales) (Dearing 1997, para. 3.84). This figure included thirty-four 'new' universities, which adopted that title after the 1992 Further and Higher Education Act, to join the forty-six 'old' universities. By 1995 total expenditure on education had reached £38 billion, compared to £28 billion in 1981 (at 1995 prices) (OPCS 1997, p. 118). There was mounting concern about the costs of higher education in particular, despite the fact that students were being asked to pay an increasing proportion of the costs of their education. Spending on higher, further and continuing education had reached £9.3 billion by 1994/5 (OPCS 1997, p. 69).

The student maintenance grant had decreased in real terms since the late 1980s. The cash value of the grant was frozen at the 1990/1 level until 1994/5, since when it has been reduced by around 10 per cent each year. Meanwhile the proportion of students taking out loans increased to 55 per cent in 1994/5, with the average amount being borrowed increasing year on year (OPCS 1997, p. 69).

By 1995/6 there was a total of 1,720,000 higher education students in the UK (HESA 1997) compared to 618,000 in 1970/1 (OPCS 1997, p. 64).

Further education

In 1995 there were 465 colleges of further education with a total of 2,607,000 part-time and full-time students (OPCS 1997, p. 64). Funding through the Training and Enterprise Councils (TECs, see Glossary) had by now become particularly important for further education, as had the national vocational qualifications framework. Colleges began concentrating on full-time students as they responded to the government's desire to increase full-time further education participation rates. This trend was reinforced by a continuing recession and the lack of apprenticeships in industry. As a result the proportion of students on day-release fell considerably (Hall 1994). Table 2.2 gives information about the types of enrolments in further education. More recent data are not strictly comparable with those in the table because of changes in definitions; however, there has been a steady increase in enrolments to further education, with a total of 2.5 million in 1997/8 (OPCS 2001, p. 65)

Adult education

Adults can enrol on a wide variety of day and evening courses: academic, vocational and leisure-oriented. Around 1.1 million adults in England and Wales were enrolled on courses in adult education centres in 1994/5 (OPCS 1997, p. 66). Additionally there are hundreds of other agencies involved in adult education, e.g. correspondence colleges, women's institutes, the Workers' Education Association and the National Extension College. Universities are now autonomous bodies responsible for managing their own curricula, assessments and finances. Adults can improve their literacy and numeracy skills by enrolling on a basic skills course. The numbers doing so increased steadily over the ten years to 1994/5, with a total of 208,000 receiving tuition in this area in England and Wales in that year (OPCS 1997, p. 67).

The situation in 2001

The Labour government was elected in 1997. At that point there was an increase in government spending on HE from £4.7 billion in 1997

Table 2.2 Enrolments on further education courses leading to a qualification: by type of course and gender, 1994/5

	Thousands			
	Full time		Part time	
	Males	Females	Males	Females
NVQs				
Level 1	13.9	6.9	40.7	26.0
Level 2	25.7	34.4	62.4	54.1
Level 3	10.0	12.7	35.0	27.8
GNVQs				
Foundation	2.2	3.4	0.3	0.9
Intermediate	22.4	22.3	1.8	2.3
Advanced	34.6	39.0	3.4	3.6
Other vocational qualifications	139.8	139.5	256.2	371.1
GCE A/AS	76.3	91.0	50.2	76.7
GCSE	13.1	11.8	50.7	88.8
All courses leading to specified qualifications	338.0	361.0	500.8	651.3
All courses leading to unspecified qualifications	30.3	27.2	222.1	430.4
All further education courses	368.3	388.3	723.0	1,081.7

Source OPCS 1997, p. 64, table 3.17

to £5.8 billion in 2001 (a real-terms increase of 18 per cent). This compares with a real-terms cut of 36 per cent over the Conservative period of office. The funding per student between 1997 and 2001 remained roughly steady. Again, even this seems favourable compared to the cut in the unit of funding (pounds per student) of 36 per cent between 1989 and 1997. However, expressed as a proportion of GDP, it declined from 0.99 to 0.96 per cent during that period of Labour office.

For students as individuals the situation deteriorated. Government spending on maintenance grants declined from £932 million to £140 million, student–staff ratios increased from 16:1 to 17:1, staff spent more of their time (around 30 per cent) preparing for teaching quality assessment exercises rather than actually teaching, and the average student debt on completing an undergraduate degree reached £2,500, a real-terms increase of almost 200 per cent over the first term of the Labour government, 1997–2001 (Thomson 2001).

Into the twenty-first century: mass higher education

The idea of a 'mass' system of higher education builds on Trow's classic formulation of elite, mass and universal systems (Trow 1970). The transition point from the first to the second occurs when the proportion of the 18–21 year olds attending HE surpasses 15 per cent. In Britain this happened in 1988 when the age participation index reached 15.1 per cent (DES 1991b). Once the figure passes 40 per cent the system evolves into its universal stage (Trow 1970).

The 1980s and 1990s saw intense and accelerating change in higher education, leaving a difficult legacy for the twenty-first century. Four main areas of change have been associated with the move to a 'mass' system in the UK: its size; changing patterns of access; a relative decline in resources and a change in the functions that higher education is expected to fulfil.

The expansion of higher education

The growth in the higher education system is the most obvious change. Some of the key data about this are as follows:

- In the thirty-two years between 1960 and 1992 the percentage of 18–21 year olds attending university increased from 6.9 per cent to 13.3 per cent in 1982 and 27.8 per cent in 1992 (DES 1991b and DfE 1994). By 2000 it had reached 33 per cent.
- The fastest period of growth occurred between the early 1980s and the early 1990s. There was a slowdown in 1993 when the funding system changed. The replacement of student grants with loans, and then the requirement for many to contribute to university fees, meant a decline in demand for higher education. There were just under seven hundred thousand home part-time and full-time students in the UK in 1988/9 (DES 1991b) compared with one and a half million in 1995/6 (HESA 1997): more than doubling in seven years, but the figure remained at around that point subsequently.

Changing Patterns of Access: gender, age, part-time students, social class, disability, ethnicity

Only 42 per cent of first-year higher education students were women in 1982, rising to 47 per cent in 1989 and staying at that figure between 1989 and 1992 (DfE 1994, p. 1). The sexes continued to be unevenly distributed around different curriculum areas. By 1994 the sexes became equally represented among first-year full-time undergraduates for the first time (HESA 1995) and stayed roughly equal thereafter. By 2001 around 55 per cent of students were women, though their distribution was heavily dependent upon subject area and type of institution.

The proportion of entrants aged between 21 and 24 years increased from 7.2 per cent in 1982 to 9.5 per cent in 1992, though it dipped to 6.4 per cent in 1990 (DfE 1994, p. 2). The proportion of new entrants aged over 25 years increased from 0.2 per cent in 1982 to 0.6 per cent in 1992, with much of the gain being made in the final two years of that period (an increase of 0.3 per cent) (ibid.). By 1992 the percentage of all students aged 21 and over in the UK was 42 per cent, compared to 33 per cent in 1982, with most of the growth occurring in the undergraduate population (DfE, 1994 table 3). By 2000 the figure had reached almost 66 per cent, and nearer 70 per cent in some post-1992 universities (HESA 2001).

The number of part-time students rose rapidly in the decade between 1982 and 1992: by 41 per cent in the Open University, by 101 per cent in other chartered universities and by 60 per cent in polytechnics and colleges, though the percentage varied considerably by level of course (HESA 1995, p. 5). By 2000/1 around 50 per cent of undergraduates were studying on a part-time basis (Office for National Statistics 2002).

The professional classes constitute 20 per cent of the population; 80 per cent of young people from these classes go on to higher education. For the least skilled only around 10 per cent go on to higher education and in no other social group does the figure exceed 50 per cent. Even when equipped with the necessary qualifications, people from the lower three of five social classes are only 70 per cent as likely to enter universities or colleges as those from the top two social groups (and they are more likely to study locally and part-time). Students from less skilled backgrounds account for only 20 per cent of students in universities established before 1992 (and many are mature students). Post-1992 universities attract 60 per cent more applications from these groups than pre-1992 universities do. Despite three years of the Labour government's widening participation policy, the number of students from unskilled backgrounds had risen by only five hundred by the year 2000: from five thousand in 1995 (Thomson 2001). However, the number of students from partly skilled backgrounds grew more steeply: from nearly two thousand to just over 24,000 in the same period. By 1999/2000, while 50,970 students of the total 113,470 came from a management, administration or professional background, only 8,240 came from plant/machine operative or sales occupations (HESA, 2001).

About 3 per cent of first-year students at all levels in the UK have a disability (HESA 1995, 1997) compared with 20 per cent of the general population who reported long-standing illness, disability or infirmity in 1993 (OPCS 1995, table 7.10, p. 21).

Using the OPCS categories and looking only at full- and part-time first-year students of known ethnicity in UK, 4.1 per cent were black, 3.2 per cent Indian, 1.6 per cent Pakistani and 4 per cent from other groups (HESA 1997, p. 184).

To summarize, then, we can say that there are more women, older students, part-time students and members of some minority ethnic groups (for example Africans, Indians, East African Asians and Chinese) in higher education than previously. Disadvantages remain, however, in terms of social class, disability and for some other minority ethnic groups (for example Bangladeshis) and there is little sign of the gap closing for these groups (Egerton and Halsey 1993; Modood 1993; Shiner and Modood 2002). Where access has improved for social groups it has tended to mean access to less prestigious institutions and qualifications.

Relative decline in resources

The increase in student numbers was not matched by an increase in public resources in the 1980s and 1990s:

- The index of public funding per full-time equivalent student between 1979 and 1989 rose from a base of 100 to 103 in the universities and fell from 100 to 75 in the polytechnics (Watson 1996). In cash terms this translates into a fall for the polytechnics from around £5,500 to just over £3,000 per student, while the university figure stayed at around £6,500 (Brookman 1992).
- There has been a dramatic decline in the relative level of resourcing provided for higher education more recently. With an index set at 100 in 1989/90 the unit of resource fell to 75 points by 1994/5 and fell to 69 by 1997/8 (Watson 1996).
- This meant an increase in student–staff ratios, rising from 9:1 to 12:1 in the universities and 8:1 to 16:1 in the polytechnics between 1982 and 1992 (Ball 1992), a reduction in resources available for research, teaching and learning and a decline in physical structure of universities themselves.
- However, looked at in absolute terms rather than relative to student numbers, spending on higher education has grown enormously: only £219 million of public money was spent per year on higher education in England, Scotland and Wales combined in the early 1960s compared to £7 billion on English universities alone in 1992/3 (Scott 1995).

One of the ways in which universities have both encouraged and coped with this under-funded expansion is to change their curriculum structure, at the same time reducing the amount of teaching time given to students. Large parts of the higher education system have adopted the model of higher education used in the United States, which had a mass system long before the UK. This system works by awarding credit for modules of study successfully passed with this credit being accumulated by the student until they have enough for a degree. Students usually study within a two-semester academic year when this model is adopted and can take advantage of other features such as the accreditation of prior learning, which makes their period of study shorter. The modular credit structure is also claimed to be more efficient than the traditional British system in other ways: generic modules can be 'delivered' to a mixed student group and a modular structure can be 'managed' centrally much more efficiently. About 80 per cent of universities had or were committed to developing modular programmes by 1994, nearly 85 per cent had or planned to introduce a credit accumulation and transfer scheme, 65 per cent had or planned to adopt a two-semester structure and 70 per cent allowed credit for work-based and other forms of experiential learning (Robertson 1994, p. 10).

Changes in the functions of higher education

Robbins (Committee on Higher Education 1963) defined the functions of higher education as including:

- instruction in occupational skills (to develop the nation's economy)
- the advancement of learning (to develop knowledge)
- promotion of the powers of the mind (to develop the intellect of the person)
- the transmission of a common culture and common standards of citizenship (to develop society).

Emphasis on the purposes of higher education tends to shift between these functions depending on the economic and political situation of the time. Beginning with the 1985 Green Paper *The Development of Higher Education into the 1990s*, which emphasized higher education contributing 'more effectively to the improvement of the performance of the economy', there has been increasing emphasis on the first of Robbins's functions and a de-emphasis on the others, particularly the last two. By 1991 government rhetoric and the funding mechanisms in place made it clear that the emphasis was now on the vocational relevance of post-compulsory education and its contribution to 'UK plc' rather than on any personal development it may involve for the individual or on the cultural and intellectual development of society. This was re-emphasized in David Blunkett's speech at Greenwich University when he was Education Secretary in 2000:

> Higher education must also equip all graduates with the skills and abilities they need to perform effectively in the workplace and build rewarding careers. The public investment in students is substantial – as indeed is the financial contribution made by students themselves. So it is critical that graduates should leave higher education able and prepared to make an early and effective contribution to the knowledge-based economy. That means possession, alongside specialist knowledge, of ICT and other key skills; a flair for enterprise; the ability to think creatively, and an understanding of the working environment.
>
> (http://cms1.gre.ac.uk/dfee/#speech,
> accessed 22 January 2002)

Critique of the expansion towards 'mass' higher education

Trow (1994) notes that the 1991 White Paper *Higher Education: A New Framework* anticipates growth yet says nothing about capital investment, discusses 'quality' and 'efficiency' yet is blind to the real value of higher education, proposes economies yet creates impoverishment. Barnett (1994), too, worries about the move from propositional knowledge, 'knowing that', towards performativity, 'knowing how', in the university sector. Whatever one's opinion of it, however, there is no doubt that the view of the key role of universities outlined in the 1991 White Paper has left its mark on institutions as a result of the funding mechanisms used by the government to achieve the desired outcomes. For Ritzer (1996) and

Jary and Parker (1995) for example there has been a 'McDonald-ization' of universities in the UK: a concern with systematized processes and managerialism which has led to increased instru-mentalism on the part of staff and students and an overall decline in the quality of higher education.

It is clear that higher education today in the UK is very different from what it was. Lecturers work harder and many have little time for research and careful thought. Students have suffered increas-ing depletion of the resources available to them and have had to bear more of the costs of their education. They are also at the sharp end of the strategies that universities have adopted to cope with increasing student numbers and fewer resources. On the positive side higher education is no longer a privilege for the elite alone. However, the important question for previously excluded groups is 'access to what?' Privileged groups are extremely good at gaining advantage in most situations and, as British higher education becomes increasingly differentiated, these groups are largely to be found in the better resourced, more prestigious institutions. In reality the system has not become a 'mass' one at all, nor even a 'crowded elite' one (Robertson, 1996). Rather it is polarizing into a mass/elite framework, and here there are clear parallels with the effect of 'parental choice' on the school system, with the increasing division between 'magnet' and 'sink' schools.

Case study: the new vocationalism

Over the course of the 1980s the government developed policies to tackle the steadily rising unemployment levels among the young. By 1986 the official figure was 12 per cent unemployed in total: 3 million people, many of them school leavers. Three factors concerned the government in this: the costs of benefits for the unemployed; the social and economic costs of unemployment; and the long-term effects on young people, particularly their employability in the future. What became known at the time as the 'new vocationalism' was seen by the New Right as a solution. It put human capital theory (Schultz 1961) into practice, the basic idea of which was that investment in human resource 'capital' through training now would yield dividends to the country later. It also attempted to strengthen the links between education and the economy. The aims of the new vocationalism were as follows.

First, vocational qualifications were to be rationalized so that employers in Britain and abroad knew what they meant. The thousands of vocational qualifications would be organized into a simple structure; holders of those qualifications would have a record of achievement which told prospective employers exactly what they were competent to do. These principles underpin both the Modern Apprenticeship scheme (see p. 57) and the setting up in 1986 of the National Council for Vocational Qualifications, which quickly established the National Vocational Qualifications (NVQ) framework. The aim of the NVQ scheme was to simplify what had been a confusing multitude of vocational courses and awards into a single coherent system of qualifications at five distinct levels. Each qualification states very explicitly what its holders can do by giving clear statements of competence which they must achieve to be awarded it. These competence statements have been formulated by industry and commerce in 'lead bodies' to ensure that they match what people need in the workplace. The qualifications are modular in design. This means that the programme of study is broken into separately assessed smaller pieces; people can achieve small sets of competences at different times, until all those required for the qualification are attained. For people with families or with shifting work patterns or other responsibilities, modular programmes are ideal, giving access to qualifications and easy part-time study. Also, people who can demonstrate that they have already got some competences can obtain certificates to prove it without needing to follow a course. In 1997 around 80 per cent of the workforce were in occupations which had NVQ qualifications.

The claimed advantages of the competence framework are the following:

- Assessment of observable performance is far more reliable than of non-observable characteristics such as knowledge and understanding. It is better, therefore, to assess behaviour than knowledge. If students can show themselves capable of carrying out specified tasks, the necessary knowledge must have been acquired and does not need to be separately assessed anyway.

- Assessment in NVQs is one-to-one and takes place only when the individual is ready. Individuals can progress through their studies at a pace appropriate to them. This is true personalized training.

- Rigorous assessment and accreditation of small elements of competence means that employers will know exactly what job applicants are capable of doing.

- Explicitly setting out units and elements of competence with associated performance criteria and range statements means that assessment is fair and objective. What is being tested is clear to all, including (and especially) the student.

- Competence statements are based on a careful functional analysis of jobs. Employers are involved in this through the lead bodies. The learning is thorough and job-related. There is neither too little nor too much learning, and it is all relevant.

- Training institutions such as colleges are paid by results (the number of students successfully gaining competence). This is known as output-related funding. It means they are motivated to achieve high-quality training so the pass rate is high and they receive more money.

- Most vocational qualifications at the lower levels have now been 'NVQd'. The NVQ approach is being applied in higher education at Levels 4 and 5. This will have all the advantages of the currently available NVQs, particularly their vocational relevance, clearly stated learning outcomes and objective assessment.

Second, education was to be vocationalized in schools, further education and adult education. Since Callaghan's 1976 Ruskin speech there had been a public articulation amongst policy-makers that the British education system was anti-vocational and that this was detrimental to Britain's competitiveness in the international economy. This aspect of the new vocationalism was oriented to injecting vocational courses into the curriculum as pupils came close to leaving school, and also aimed at giving them an understanding of and enthusiasm for industry and commerce. The Technical and Vocational Education Initiative (TVEI, see Glossary) is one example of how this was done.

Third, the unemployed were to be trained for work, giving them 'key skills' (now defined as information technology, numeracy and communication) and a record of achievement in the process. Government policy increasingly turned to training for unemployed young people, rather than simply the payment of benefits. A sequence of schemes for the young was the consequence: the Youth Opportunities Programme; the Youth Training Scheme; Youth Training; Employment Training and so on.

Fourth, the quality of vocational education and training was to be improved. Here policy measures were designed to improve both the status and the content of vocational education and training. One of the ways of achieving this was through the development of training credits. Underpinning this policy measure was a set of neo-liberal ideas concerning the 'marketization' of vocational education and training. If young people were given what appeared to be a cheque or credit card, with a value of around £1,000 to spend on their training, then they would become selective consumers and the providers would have to ensure that they offered top-quality training provision in order to attract them.

The critique of new vocationalism

A number of criticisms of the policies associated with new vocationalism have been made by academics. They include the following.

• Policy was concentrated on the lower levels of education and training and on lower achievers, rather than areas of the economy which would make British industry competitive abroad. Roger Dale's (1985b) study concluded that YT and similar schemes were aimed at lower-ability 14–18 year olds and trained them for very low-skilled, insecure employment. Hence, rather than training them for employment, these schemes prepared them for a status somewhere between work and non-work; they did not address the real needs of the country for high-level skills. Peter Robinson's study concluded that NVQs:

are heavily concentrated in the clerical and secretarial and the personal service and sales occupations, and in the (internationally) sheltered service sectors of the economy. They are under-represented in the higher managerial, professional and technical occupations, in the craft occupations, and in the (internationally) exposed manufacturing and business and financial services sectors of the economy.

(Robinson 1996, p. 34)

- Training has not enhanced social mobility for individuals and groups undertaking it; rather it has tended to reproduce existing social inequalities based, for example, on race and gender. Gleeson concludes that:

> in the specific case of female participation in nursing, child care and other gender-specific courses . . . vocational training represents little more than a reinforcement in gender roles and apprenticeship in home crafts . . . [while] evidence regarding black youth on [YT] courses indicates that they are consistently more likely to be allocated to schemes offering inferior opportunities of subsequent employment.

(Gleeson 1989, p. 29)

David Lee and his co-researchers found much the same thing in their study (1990, pp. 121–3).

- These policies have sometimes not achieved even their basic aims, and have cost considerable amounts of money to set up and monitor. Peter Robinson (1996) concludes that the NCVQ framework has not rationalized the overall structure of qualifications as was its intention. Awards of traditional vocational qualifications in 1994–5 were still significantly higher than awards of NVQs (and GNVQs), and there was by 1995 a wider array of qualifications than was the case before the introduction of NVQs. He estimates that around £107 million was spent directly on setting up the framework, with additional costs for publicity and staff time.
- Much 'training' has in fact been preparation for unemployment. Training schemes are simply a way of making the unemployment figures smaller and less politically damaging. Even one of the Conservative government's own ministers, Alan Clark, when Minister of State at the Department of Employment, became

convinced that this was the case. As he wrote in his diary in June 1983: 'a mass of "schemes" whose purpose, plainly, is not so much to bring relief to those out of work as to devise excuses for removing them from the [unemployment] Register' (Clark 1993, pp. 9–10).

- New vocational policies have shifted power into the hands of employers and national politicians. Teachers, lecturers, parents, students and the local community have lost control of education and training. Professions too have lost their autonomy as a result of central control of professional qualifications (Jones and Moore 1993). Industrial and commercial 'lead bodies' set the competences for NVQs, for example, largely excluding the former groups from control over 'syllabuses'. Even within the lead bodies more powerful, larger, companies have exercised control (Eraut et al. 1996, pp. 2–4).

- While there has been a rash of vocational education and training initiatives, these have often been short-lived and have worked in isolation. The changes from the Youth Opportunities Programme to the Youth Training Scheme and its variants are one example of this. At each twist of policy, schemes came to an abrupt halt, staff were made unemployed and young people faced insecurity about their next step.

- The political nature of policy-making has resulted in confused and changing policies with too many unclear aims. In the area of higher education, the changing policies on funding have meant that universities and other institutions have found planning extremely difficult. Developing the facilities to accommodate increased student numbers takes time. Many institutions have found that by the time they have committed funds to building programmes for student accommodation and teaching facilities, policy has changed, increasing student numbers have attracted financial penalties and the overall unit of resource (funding per student) has been cut. In the post-compulsory sector in general this has caused severe financial difficulties for many institutions, with consequent effects in the quality of their provision, staff redundancies and so on.

- There are numerous criticisms of the teaching and learning principles underlying the whole competence-based approach (e.g.

see Ashworth and Saxton 1990). Though the details of this are not relevant here, it seems that government policy may be based on an inaccurate or inappropriate theoretical base.

- Output-related funding has tempted colleges to pass students who would otherwise fail. BTEC (Business and Technician Education Council) became aware of this happening in 1994 and had to increase its monitoring of standards. Lecturers knew it was happening but could not say anything for fear of losing their jobs.

- While a competence-based approach may be appropriate for the lower levels of training, where observable skills are more important, transfer to higher levels is very difficult and may actually lower standards. Since NVQs were first applied to the lower levels, this was not immediately apparent; but as attempts are made to make Levels 4 and 5 competence-based it is becoming increasingly obvious. Between the years 1990/1 and 1994/5 there was no growth in the number of NVQ awards at Level 3 and a fall in the number of awards at the two highest levels, 4 and 5 (Robinson 1996, p. 34).

Key points

- Governments have increasingly viewed post-compulsory education in terms of its relevance for the economy and have attempted to steer it in a vocational direction in recent years.

- Policies often have unintended outcomes, as was shown to be the case with several aspects of the 'new vocationalism' of the 1980s.

- Policy-making in the area of post-compulsory policy since 1979 has been less coherent than policy in the area of compulsory education. In the latter there is a clear progression in policy-making from 1980 onwards (as we saw in Chapter 1). The post-compulsory area is marked by changes in policy content (e.g. encouraging expansion of higher education or restricting it) and in the role of government, from dirigisme (the cuts of the early 1980s) to laissez-faire (the unregulated expansion of the later 1980s and early 1990s), back to dirigisme from the Autumn Statement of 1993.

- The dilemma of how to pay for expanded post-compulsory provision has been a key policy issue since the rapid expansion of higher education in the mid-1980s. Governments have been content to allow the relatively disadvantaged status and resourcing of further and adult education students to persist.

Guide to further reading

For a good overview of the further education sector see:

Cantor, L., Roberts, I. and Pratley, B. (1995) *A Guide to Further Education in England and Wales*, London: Cassell.

Hall, V. (1994) *Further Education in the United Kingdom*, London: Collins Educational/Staff College.

For an interesting account of the implementation of youth training schemes see:

Lee, D., Marsden, D., Rickman, P. and Duncombe, J. (1990) *Scheming for Youth*, Buckingham: Open University Press.

For a discussion of the changing shape of higher education see:

Scott, P. (1995) *The Meanings of Mass Higher Education*, Buckingham: Open University Press/SRHE.

Warner, D. and Palfreyman, D. (2001) *The State of UK Higher Education: Managing Change and Diversity*, Buckingham: Open University Press/SRHE.

For an insight see:

Halsey, A. H. (1992) *Decline of Donnish Dominion*, Oxford: Oxford University Press.

This traces the development of what Halsey considers to be the current crisis in higher education. Halsey considers that the system is now too bureaucratic and is under-funded, while at the same time the position of the academic in British society has been undermined. Halsey's survey of academics, the most recent in a series he has conducted over the years, reveals a situation of low morale, disappointment and decline. The book provides a good background to reading and thinking about the implications of the 1997 Dearing Report (see Chapter 5).

Useful addresses

Literature on a number of areas of government policy in the vocational education and training (VET) area is available from:
Department for Education and Skills
Most of the Department's publications can be ordered through:
PROLOG
PO BOX 5050
Sherwood Park
Annesley
Notts
NG15 ODJ
www.dfes.gov.uk/publications

Reports on Vocational Education and Training in Further Education can be obtained from:
Learning and Skills Development Agency
Sales and Marketing Team
Tel: 020 7297 9123
email: registrations@lsda.org.uk
www.lsda.org.uk

Useful websites

http://www.hefce.ac.uk/
The home page of the Higher Education Funding Council for England.
The site for the Welsh funding councils is at www.wfc.ac.uk and for Scotland at www.shefc.ac.uk

http://www.thesis.co.uk/
The web service of the *Times Higher Education Supplement*

http://www.universitiesuk.ac.uk/
The home page of Universities UK: the organization of university vice-chancellors and principals

http://www.srhe.ac.uk/srhe
The home page of the Society for Research into Higher Education

http://www.niss.ac.uk/
The gateway to many education-related sites, including most university library catalogues in the UK

http://www.thebiz.co.uk/
Allows you to search for details of institutions and other information to do with training and development in the UK

http://www.lsda.ac.uk/
The Learning and Skills Development Agency's website, containing details and text of their publications and other useful information about further education

http://www.qaa.ac.uk/
The website of the Quality Assurance Agency, which aims to promote confidence in the quality and standards within higher education

http://www.ucisa.ac.uk/
The website of the Universities and Colleges Information Systems Association, giving much useful information about post-compulsory education and access to other websites, including a powerful search engine

http://www.edexcel.org.uk/
The home page of Edexcel: the 'foundation for educational excellence'. Edexcel is an amalgation of BTEC and London Examinations, one of the examination boards. A range of information about training and development and examinations, among other things, is available here

http://www.lifelonglearning.co.uk
The website for the encouragement, promotion and development of lifelong learning

Chapter 3
Making education policy

OUTLINE
This chapter explores the nature of education policy and seeks
to give some insight into the policy-making process. It begins by
asking the apparently simple question 'what is education
policy?' and then goes on to explore the ways in which it is
made, concentrating on the national level (although education
policy is explicitly or implicitly made wherever there is an
educative process). Two case studies are provided to show in
some detail how policy was made, first, in the area of schools
being allowed to opt out of local authority control and, second,
in the development of the national curriculum. The discussion
then moves on to some conceptual tools for understanding the
forces that drive the policy-making process, particularly the
political and educational ideologies which provide guidance for
action. Finally, an attempt is made to show that, although there
is often a clear link between ideology and policy, the relationship
between them is very frequently mediated by a number of other
less predictable factors. Some illustrations of these are given.

What is education policy?

Education policy is often thought of as a *thing*: a statement of some
sort, usually written down in a policy document. Viewed in this way,
education policy could be defined as follows:

> a specification of principles and actions, related to educational
> issues, which are followed or which should be followed and
> which are designed to bring about desired goals

In this sense policy is a piece of paper, a statement of intentions or
of practice as it is perceived by policy-makers or as they would like
it to be.

This view of policy is a very limited one. It is better to see policy as a process, something which is dynamic rather than static. This dynamism comes from a number of sources:

- There is usually conflict among those who make policy, as well as those who put it into practice, about what the important issues or problems for policy are and about the desired goals.
- Interpreting policy is an active process: policy statements are almost always subject to multiple interpretations depending upon the standpoints of the people doing the interpretative 'work'.
- The practice of policy on the ground is extremely complex, both that being 'described' by policy and that intended to put policy into effect. Simple policy descriptions of practice do not capture its multiplicity and complexity, and the implementation of policy in practice almost always means outcomes differ from policy-makers' intentions (which were, anyway, always multiple and often contradictory).

Ball takes these concerns into account when he says this about policy:

> Policy is both text and action, words and deeds, it is what is enacted as well as what is intended. Policies are always incomplete insofar as they relate to or map on to the 'wild profusion' of local practice.
>
> (Ball 1994c, p. 10)

Figure 3.1 illustrates the complex nature of policy-making and interpretation.

How is education policy made?

Rein (1983, p. 211) argues that three basic steps are involved in policy-making at the national level:

- problem (or issue) setting
- the 'mobilization of the fine structure of government action'
- the 'achievement of settlements [compromises which establish a framework for policy and practice] in the face of dilemmas and trade-offs among values'.

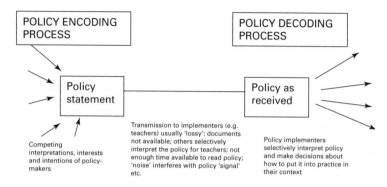

Figure 3.1 Policy encoding and decoding

Wherever policy is being made, in schools, counties or at the national level, these three steps are important: a problem is identified, the policy-making process is put into gear and the political process begins.

Using Rein's three steps we can say the following about education policy-making in Britain.

Problem/issue setting: Defining something that needs to be done is usually the work of more than one agency. Sometimes the civil service is important in highlighting an issue, sometimes a think tank such as the Institute for Economic Affairs, sometimes the press and television, and sometimes an individual such as the Prime Minister. Usually it is a combination of these. It was noted in Chapter 1, however, that teachers and the local education authorities, who had been influential in all stages of policy-making in the past, were progressively excluded from these processes during the 1980s.

The mobilization of the fine structure of government (or other agency) action: What form this takes will depend on the nature of the policy being discussed and the context of policy-making (government, school, local education authority, etc.). The two case studies below illustrate the different ways in which the policy-making process can occur at the national level.

The achievement of settlements in the face of dilemmas and trade-offs among values: Even though some important players in the policy-making process had been excluded, education policy-making remained a complex, non-linear process in the 1980s, as it continues to be today. Policies are always the product of compromises between multiple agendas and influences (Ball 1994c, p. 16). The actual outcome, the policy as articulated, will be the result of a micropolitical process and 'muddling through'.

Policy-making in practice, then, is usually far from the rational-purposive model that many people imagine it to be: one in which a distinct set of policy-makers consider sensible policies in a logical way and carefully formulate them with a clear purpose in mind. Bleiklie notes, for example, that frequently policy is far from simply 'the mechanical application of means [by the policy architect or engineer] in order to realise given ends' (Bleiklie 2000, pp. 54–5). Instead the process of 'encoding' policy is a complex one in which policy texts are developed as a process of negotiation, compromise and the exercise of power. As a result these policy texts are usually laden with multiple agendas, attitudes, values and sets of meaning. Policy encoding thus involves complex practices of interpreting, negotiating and refining proposals. The consequence is that 'processes of change at the level of national policy, within academic institutions and disciplinary groups, are only partially co-ordinated' (Kogan et al. 2000, p. 30).

Two case studies of policy-making

To illustrate and clarify how policy is made at the national level (the 'fine structure of government action'), it is useful to look in detail at some case studies. Although the cases chosen here may not be typical, especially as they both come from the school sector only, they do give important insights into the policy process in two key areas of Conservative education policy-making in the 1980s.

The first study concerns the policy which led to the creation of grant-maintained (GM) schools: schools allowed to 'opt out' of control by the local education authority to become virtually independent state schools which, in England, receive their money direct from the national Funding Agency for Schools (FAS).

The second relates to the policy process through which the national curriculum was developed, that is the schemes of study and related patterns of assessment which most children between the ages of 5 and 16 years in the English and Welsh state schooling system must follow.

Case study: policy-making on grant-maintained schools

The idea for schools opting out of local authority control to GM status came originally from Kenneth Baker, the Secretary of State for Education at the time (the mid-1980s). It fitted neatly with his desire to increase parental choice of schools, to differentiate schools more clearly in order to provide more alternatives for parents and to undermine the power of the local education authorities, to which the Conservatives were hostile. The idea was to permit individual schools to leave the control of their LEA if the majority of parents agreed to this, and for these schools to receive funding from a national agency, the FAS, so that they would become almost self-governing, while remaining in the state sector.

The civil servants in the DES had to respond to this proposal, but they were presented only with the germ of an idea, a 'sketchy policy' in the words of one civil servant, because neither Baker nor Prime Minister Margaret Thatcher really knew how the idea of opting out would work in practice. At this point the proposal entered the 'policy loop': the series of meetings between ministers and civil servants at which policy is progressively refined. One civil servant described the process in the following way.

> What we did was to take different aspects of the policy and then work up proposals and options on those. When we had something that constituted a reasonable package we put that up to ministers . . . We then had a discussion with them and they commented on various aspects with us. Then we went away and got on with it. On some occasions it might be a couple of times a week. At other times, we might be doing a substantial amount of work in between and it would be perhaps three to four weeks.
>
> (quoted in Fitz and Halpin 1991, p. 138)

Ministers rarely wrote anything during this period; they either agreed with what had been developed or asked for alternative approaches.

The interpersonal and interactive nature of the policy loop provided an opportunity for civil servants to feed a 'departmental view' into the formulation of policy, although proposals stemming from this were sometimes vetoed by ministers. For example, by insisting that the chance for GM status should be given only to schools with more than three hundred pupils, the DES effectively limited the application of the policy to middle and secondary schools (although in 1990 the government extended the possibility of GM status to all primary schools). This kind of policy input from the civil service, and the conflicts with politicians that can sometimes arise from it, was cleverly satirized in the television programmes *Yes Minister* and *Yes Prime Minister*.

This example shows that even though the original idea for GM schools came from a politician, civil servants were able to guide the policy process as they converted a sketchy outline into a workable policy. Determining the fine detail of policy on specific issues, such as parental ballots, funding of GM schools, what should be taught in them and so on, gave civil servants a good degree of power. This was possibly even more true given the exclusion of the 'educational establishment' (teachers' associations, LEAs, etc.) from the policy loop, which became increasingly restricted during the 1980s.

Case study: national curriculum policy-making

The origins of the national curriculum largely lie in the perceptions, within government and the population at large, that teachers were failing the country. The dominant image during the early 1980s was of a profession in the grip of progressivist theories of education which were resulting in generations of illiterate children. Teachers, it was believed, allowed children to follow their own interests in an unfocused way; pupils studied 'topics' rather than 'subjects' and were allowed to spend too much time off-task, chatting with friends in groups rather than listening to the teacher. Additionally, teachers were not sufficiently concerned with fitting children for life and work after school.

In the Conservative Party such criticisms were common; they were analysed and discussed in right-wing think tanks and informal groups of right-wing intellectuals, e.g. by Brian Cox and the other authors of the *Black Papers* published between 1969 and 1977 (see Cox and Dyson (eds) 1969a and b), and more recently within a variety of New-Right think tanks, such as the Centre for Policy Studies (CPS), the National Council for Educational Standards, the Social Affairs Unit, the Adam Smith Institute, the Hillgate Group and the Institute of Economic Affairs (IEA).

These groups, with the support of Margaret Thatcher, were moving towards a policy involving a minimalist national curriculum concentrating very heavily on literacy, science and numeracy. This worried many, particularly in the Department of Education and Science. Duncan Graham, who was to become Chairman and Chief Executive of the National Curriculum Council (NCC), argued that:

> somebody . . . in government or in the Education Department . . . decided to head off that group from leading state education to total disaster by inventing the national curriculum which appeared to satisfy a lot of their demands.
>
> (Graham 1993, p. 6)

Together the NCC and the School Examination and Assessment Council (SEAC) were charged with fleshing out the curriculum which became mandatory in 1988. These bodies were set up against the desires of the civil service, which wanted to have control of the curriculum. As a result they found their work undermined by some senior civil servants. Again, the education establishment was largely excluded from the policy loop.

> The Education Act reforms were not born of these people [education professionals], they were not consulted about them, indeed the government considered them to be the enemy.
>
> (Graham 1993, pp. 12–13)

The fifteen or so members of the NCC working groups were asked to determine the details of the curriculum in each of the ten subjects. Many members of these groups were appointed for their political and educational leanings. They were given only a few months to determine the whole content of the curriculum, detailing what children should know and be able to do at the ages of 7, 11, 14 and 16 years. Proposals were circulated to schools and other educational institutions, but deadlines for replies were tight: proposals were sent in the summer months when teachers were on holiday. What replies were received appear to have had very limited influence; few subsequent changes were detectable. This work was so tightly controlled by the civil service that Graham had to arrange a virtually clandestine meeting with the minister, Kenneth Baker, away from their eyes and ears, to discuss issues which he, correctly, thought Baker was not being told about (Graham 1993, p. 21).

Not everything, however, went the government's or the civil servants' way. Despite the appointment of Brian Cox, the author of some of the *Black Papers*, to chair the English working group, that group did not propose a curriculum which politicians on the right wanted. Instead of stressing grammar, spelling and the 'correct' use of English, the group (including Cox) emphasized the importance of imagination and creativity in writing, and the variety of spoken and written English forms. Neither Baker nor (particularly) Thatcher was happy. A compromise was reached, but Baker insisted that only Key Stage 1 (English up to the age of 7 years) should be implemented. This left room for further discussion about the English curriculum which, in 1993, blew up into a confrontation with the profession on the following issues:

- the central prescription of set books (and what they should be)
- whether to permit the use of class and regional dialects as against 'standard English'
- the relative merits of grammar and spelling as against imagination and creativity
- the study of modern writers as against dead ones
- the roles of critical and analytical abilities as against the appreciation of 'great writing'.

Teachers threatened to refuse to set and assess tests if the proposed Key Stage 3 (tested at 14 years) English curriculum was imposed. They were successful in gaining some compromise (a 'settlement') on these issues.

The outcome of the detailed policy-making on the national curriculum was a large, heavily prescribed set of ten subjects with a very heavy assessment workload. Everything was centrally determined, including schemes of work, what the children should know and be able to do at each stage, the format and content of testing, etc. Only the actual teaching methods were left to the teachers' discretion. Government control of these would later come to be tackled through teacher-training policy, as set out in the 1994 Education Act. The Conservatives' emphasis on traditional educational values was enshrined in the curriculum:

* an emphasis on admiration rather than analysis in English
* an emphasis on ancient rather than contemporary history
* an emphasis on subjects rather than topics
* an emphasis on rigorous conformity to grammatical and other rules rather than creativity.

The national curriculum was so 'traditional' in nature that Stephen Ball refers to it as the 'curriculum of the dead' (Ball 1990a), and Ivor Goodson identifies very strong similarities between the 1988 curriculum and the Secondary Regulations of 1904 (Goodson 1990). Moreover, the curriculum was so overloaded with content and teachers were so ground down with work, much of it assessment and bureaucratic form-filling rather than teaching, that the 1993 Dearing Report had to recommend the slimming down of content and of testing.

Understanding policy-making

In looking at the policy-making process it is useful to be clear about the ideologies which drive both policy-makers and those who put policy into practice. 'Ideology' is used here to mean:

> a framework of values, ideas and beliefs about the way society is and should be organised and about how resources should be allocated to achieve what is desired. This framework acts as a guide and a justification for behaviour.
>
> (adapted from Hartley 1983, pp. 26–7)

In education two sets of ideological forces are at work: political ideology and educational ideology.

The political ideologies at work in contemporary Britain are summarized in Table 3.1. Marxist and other radical political ideologies are not discussed here because of the limited impact they have had on postwar education policy-making.

The New Right

The New Right can most usefully be seen as an amalgam of neo-liberalism and neo-conservatism (Gamble 1988, pp. 28–9). Essentially it characterizes a political grouping more than a coherent political ideology itself. Some people think of Thatcherism and the New Right as being synonymous, but Thatcher's ideological position leaned heavily towards the neo-liberal strand of the New Right. As well as the internal division between neo-liberalism and neo-conservatism within the New Right, a number of other contradictions surround the concept (Ball 1990a, p. 41), including the following:

- The 'solid' sounding term actually represents a loose aggregation of points of view.
- Again, the solidity of the term creates the illusion that we can 'read off' education policy from 'New Right' ideology. Policy-making is more complex than that, as this chapter demonstrates.
- Policy derives from other sources than political ideology, including educational ideology, pragmatism, negotation and compromise.

The two strands of New Right thinking are inherently contradictory, as Table 3.2 demonstrates: on the left are the key issues for neo-liberalism in declining order of importance, while on the right are those for neo-conservatism, also in declining order of importance. Note how one is the inverse of the other, both in representing opposites and in their order of priority: the individual versus the nation; freedom of choice versus hierarchy and subordination and so on.

Table 3.3 shows the link between the key issues of New Right ideology and specific education policy.

Educational ideology and policy-making

Sets of values and attitudes which relate particularly to the nature of education and the educational process are also important in education policy-making. Table 3.4 sets out the nature of educational ideologies operating in contemporary Britain. The fourth educational ideology, social reconstructionism, is linked to more radical political ideologies, such as Marxism and feminism, that have so far had almost no influence in education policy-making in the UK, at least at the national level.

Table 3.5 shows the linkage between the political and the educational ideologies described in Tables 3.1 and 3.4.

Some contradictions and gaps in the ideology–policy link

The account above might suggest to the reader that policy and ideology are linked in a clear and smooth way: that education policy can be 'read off' the ideologies of politicians and others involved in policy-making. As indicated in Chapter 1, this rational model of policy-making is rarely found in reality, even during the 1980s when many of the groups and influences which were previously involved in policy-making had been excluded. Political conflict, compromise and 'muddling through' still took place.

> Old conservative . . . interests are at odds with new, manufacturing capital with finance capital, the Treasury with the DTI [Department of Trade and Industry], the neo-liberals with the neo-conservatives, wets with drys, Elizabeth House with Number 10, the DES with itself, Conservative Central Office with the Shires.
>
> (Ball 1990a, p. 19)

In addition, policy is sometimes made almost accidentally or as a result of political necessity. Ideology becomes less important in these circumstances. The independence of further education colleges, for example, came about partly by accident. The government faced a local authority funding crisis caused partly by its disastrous

Table 3.1 Political ideologies

Name	Key principles	The principles applied to education	Education policy examples
Neo-liberalism	■ The free market should be left to its own liberalism devices with the very minimum of government intervention (the provision of a police force, army and a few basic services). ■ Attempts at social planning are doomed to failure because of the complexities of society and because of the basic selfishness of people. ■ Institutions such as schools and LEAs, initially set up to serve the community, end up serving themselves ('producer capture'). ■ Institutions such as LEAs are not needed to offer strategic direction, because the 'hidden hand' of the market will ensure that the system operates for the common good.	■ Schools should compete with schools, individual pupils against each other. ■ Parents are consumers in this context and should be given the information they need to make intelligent choices. ■ Diversity within the education system should be encouraged in order to provide extensive choice: grant-maintained schools, city technology colleges, and support for the private sector can sustain this choice.	The Conservative government justified the scheme to give nursery vouchers worth around £1,000 to parents to 'spend' on the nursery of their choice in terms of 'enhanced parental control over the use of public funds to pay for education' (Conservative Research Department 1996, p. 1). Underpinning this statement are neo-liberal ideas about the importance of market forces in delivering good-quality education, in particular the beliefs that: ■ giving free rein to market forces with minimal state intervention will bring about an improvement in standards and provision: 'Vouchers for the provision of education . . . emphasise freedom of choice for parents . . . The scheme

- This is an individualist (or anti-collectivist) ideology; it sees the individual pursuing his or her own interests as the key to happiness for all. This notion was behind Thatcher's famous comment that 'there is no such thing as society' (*Woman's Own*, 31 October 1987).

- will increase the supply of places over time, extend choice for parents and require all providers taking part to work to consistent educational standards (Conservative Research Department 1996, p. 3).

- giving the opportunity to private providers of nursery education will lead to more and better provision. The Conservatives were pleased that by June 1996 over 630 private and voluntary nursery education providers had joined the scheme (Conservative Research Department 1996, p. 7).

- giving more choice to parents as consumers will push standards up: 'The vouchers give parents the enhanced power to choose a place that better suits their child's needs and to insist on high standards. They will increasingly allow parents who are not satisfied with the standards provided for their children to go elsewhere' (Conservative Research Department 1996, p. 3).

continued

Table 3.1 continued

Name	Key principles	The principles applied to education	Education policy examples
Neo-conservatism	■ Sees people as greedy, selfish and criminally inclined. ■ The government has a duty to intervene in what would otherwise be a war of each against all to ensure that morality and the social order are maintained. ■ 'Custom', 'tradition' and 'order' are key words. Central control is stressed and there is suspicion of power in local government for example and of people's freedom to choose. ■ Neo-conservatives believe in the state providing strong direction from the centre, rather than the localized and pluralistic 'referee' role for it envisaged in social democratic ideology.	'If pupils are to make the most of [the opportunity that schools offer] they must attend school regularly, and be given a clear moral lead by the governing body, the head teacher and the staff of their schools. Pupils must be helped to recognise their responsibilities to themselves and to others' (Department for Education 1992)	The neo-conservative influence is evident in national curriculum policy, particularly in the following features: ■ its centralism: the curriculum was determined at the national level and imposed on schools ■ its emphasis on conformity and order: common standards for all, regardless of background and region, were imposed ■ its stress on British nationhood: the curriculum tends to concentrate on British history and on English writers ■ its emphasis on the past rather than on the present and the future: this is why Ball calls it 'the curriculum of the dead' ■ its emphasis on testing, ranking and sorting

Social democracy

- There is a need for intervention by state agencies into most aspects of social provision, including education.
- Working with charitable and private agencies is acceptable, as these complement the work of the state if properly supported and regulated.
- Without regulation social inequalities will become exacerbated and the disadvantaged will become relatively, and in some cases absolutely, worse off.
- Social democrats tend to believe in the importance of pluralistic decision-making, with key players (teachers' associations, LEAs, parents, business) all being involved at both the national and local levels in matters which affect them.

- Education is an important means by which social inequality can be both mitigated and made more meritocratic.
- An educated society can deliver improved economic performance nationally; that education leads to greater levels of social mobility based on merit, particularly intelligence and hard work.
- State intervention is necessary to achieve a key goal of equality of opportunity. This is defined in terms of the ability of each individual and social group to achieve their full potential, unrestricted by limitations imposed by socio-economic background, prejudice or discrimination.

The Labour government rejected the nursery voucher scheme, arguing that 'this reliance on the market instead of a planned expansion of provision means that the government cannot offer a guarantee of a place for all four year olds' (Labour Party 1997, p. 2). Labour used the same amount of money to open new places allocated by the Conservatives for the voucher scheme: 'We will build on current provision, working with all the partners in pre-school education – LEAs, playgroups, private and voluntary sector providers' (Labour Party 1997, p. 4). This stressed strategy and planning, instead of market forces, and an increased role for the state in order to achieve objectives. Also important in this statement is the idea of consultation with interested parties rather than simply giving power to 'consumers'.

continued

Table 3.1 continued

Name	Key principles	The principles applied to education	Education policy examples
Social democracy (continued)			■ The provision of early education in nurseries is considered to be extremely important for the larger society and for mitigating social disadvantage: 'Half of a child's educational development is believed to take place in the first five years of life. Early childhood education is of great benefit to children, their families and society at large . . . Recent research by the Audit Commission found that nursery education had a clear positive effect on pupils, more than compensating for the effect of coming from a disadvantaged background' (Labour Party 1997, p. 1). ■ National and local government intervention and planning complemented by the guided

work of private and charitable institutions, not market forces, is the best way to deliver nursery education: 'We will expect LEAs to draw up development plans for the under fives, in conjunction with private and voluntary sector providers, setting out a local strategy towards meeting our pledge for all three and four year olds' (Labour Party 1997, p. 4).

■ Equality of opportunity is fostered by clear objectives and planning for nursery education: 'Studies in the United States show that children who experienced pre-school education did better in school, stayed in education longer, were more likely to gain jobs and were less likely to show delinquent behaviour ... Early years education offers an excellent opportunity to identify, at the earliest possible moment, children who have special educational needs' (Labour Party 1997, p. 1).

Table 3.2 The contradictory strands in New Right thinking

Neo-liberalism		Neo-conservatism
The individual		Strong government
Freedom of choice	Declining	Social authoritarianism
Market society	importance	Disciplined society
Laissez-faire		Hierarchy and subordination
▼ Minimal government		▼ The nation

poll tax policy, which was expensive to administer and difficult to collect. One way of solving this problem and making the poll tax appear to work was by removing colleges from council budgets. In the end, however, the poll tax was changed, but colleges remained independent.

Another factor is the difficulty of making policies that will work; understanding causes and effects in the social world is extremely complex and 'solutions' are not easy to find. Conservative government policy on training was often incoherent and self-defeating. Measures designed to save money, for example, actually turned out to cost more than previous policy. National curriculum assessment on its own cost £469 million between 1988 and 1992, with £35 million spent on virtually unused tests in 1993 (Lawton 1994, p. 103). The nursery vouchers scheme – a government scheme to support the costs of nursery care through giving vouchers to parents of young children – proved to be extremely expensive to administer, bureaucratic in operation and had rather limited effects. In fact in some areas nurseries began to close as schools extended their provision to take advantage of the scheme.

Perhaps the most important cause of the complex and contradictory nature of education policy during the 1980s and 1990s, however, was the inherently paradoxical nature of New Right thinking. Some examples follow.

The centralization–deregulation paradox

The neo-conservative desire to centralize education policy-making and control is in opposition to the neo-liberal desire to increase choice and stimulate market forces. Thus simultaneously neo-liberal

Table 3.3 New Right ideology and educational policy
See the Glossary and chapters 1 and 2 for more details of these policies.

Neo-liberal thinking	Policy example
The individual	*Parents' charter*: sets out individual parental rights and responsibilities. *Statutory publication of examination results*: gives individual parents the information on which to base school choice.
Freedom of choice	*Parental choice of schools*: parents no longer directed by LEA as to which school their child should go to. *Diversity of schools*: new types of schools developed and schools encouraged to establish unique 'mission' so that there is diversity of choice.
Market society	*Competition between schools*: schools encouraged by financial carrots and sticks to compete for pupils. *Nursery and training vouchers*: parents and students encouraged to 'shop around' for education by having vouchers to spend.
Laissez-faire	*Private schools*: allowed to thrive alongside the state system. *New universities*: given powers to accredit their own courses without oversight by national body (the CNAA).
Minimal government	*Reduced role of LEAs*: powers taken away with regard to opted out schools, colleges of further education and new universities; even maintained schools have more financial control under LMS.

continued

Table 3.3 *continued*

Neo-conservative thinking	Policy example
Strong government	*The national curriculum* imposed from the centre.
Social authoritarianism	*Stress on cultural heritage* in curriculum rather than cultural analysis.
Disciplined society	*Use of standard English* in schools rather than allowing diversity in class and regional dialects.
	Traditional approaches to teaching stressed with teacher at the front of disciplined and quiet class.
Hierarchy and subordination	*League tables and testing* create hierarchies among schools.
	Streaming of pupils in schools creates internal hierarchies.
The nation	*Nationalistic content of national curriculum* stresses parochialism rather than internationalism.

policy, such as local management of schools and opting out to grant-maintained status, is combined with a national curriculum which all state schools must follow and which initially allowed no space for anything else. Moreover, this was a national curriculum founded on at least a rhetorical stress on the 3Rs: 'back to basics' and 'market choice' make curious bedfellows. Overall the very strong centralization of policy-making in the years of Conservative government combined with increasing levels of control placed in the hands of the Secretary of State despite a rhetorical concern with devolving powers to schools and parents (as consumers).

Table 3.4 Educational ideologies

Educational ideology	Key points	Policy examples
Traditionalism	■ Traditionalism is rooted in a belief in the value of a cultural and disciplinary heritage, of which academics are custodians. The role of schools is to transmit this heritage to the next generation who are expected to receive it passively and gratefully. ■ Elitism is justified in terms of the inherent difficulties of achieving a good education and limited distribution of talent in society. ■ The content of subjects is vitally important: learning about history, geography and the rest is important in itself and helps develop the mind and personality. ■ Teachers are custodians of a great heritage.	The Education Secretary's comments on the 'Three Wise Men' report *Curriculum Organization and Classroom Practice in Primary Schools*, 1992: In responding to this government-commissioned report the Education Secretary stressed the following: ■ its critique of progressivist techniques found in schools (group work, discussion, etc.) ■ too much concentration on 'topics' rather than 'subjects' in primary schools – this often meant just copying from books ■ the over-reluctance of teachers to tell pupils things – progressivist ideology wrongly encouraged them to ask questions and elicit information rather than tell. Didactic approaches are often better than discovery learning ■ an over-emphasis on equality of opportunity, resulting in the fear of being 'elitist'. This has lowered standards.

continued

Table 3.4 *continued*

Educational ideology	Key points	Policy examples
Progressivism	■ Progressivism claims to be 'student-centred', in the sense of valuing students' participation in planning, delivering, assessing and evaluating courses. ■ Disciplinary knowledge and traditions are considered to be relatively unimportant: students' freedom of choice and personal development take priority over subject knowledge. ■ This ideology rejects elitism and favours mass access in higher education. Where there is concern about social inequality the role of education is to give a 'step up' to disadvantaged individuals and groups in the largest numbers possible, not to reconstruct society.	The Plowden Report (1968) is often used as an example of progressivism. It recommended that: ■ teachers and parents should be partners in the educational process ■ streaming in schools has deleterious effects and should be stopped ■ time should be given to children for imaginative and expressive work ■ books used and topics taught should make sense to children, and teachers need to understand the child's point of view.
Enterprise	■ Education is primarily concerned with developing people to be good and efficient workers. ■ 'What will it help us to do?' is the key question in deciding what should be taught. ■ New technology and new approaches to teaching and learning are valued both as more efficient and more effective tools than	The *Education and Training for the Twenty First Century* White Paper (1991) put forward: ■ the proposal to extend the educational voucher in the form of a 'training credit' with which young people could buy vocational training ■ a philosophy of adult education which would lead to funding only where it is vocationally relevant or caters for adults with special

traditional approaches, and for their development of important skills in students.

■ There is considerable emphasis on 'core skills': communication, IT, literacy, etc.

educational needs. Non-vocational adult education would lose funding

■ the proposal that colleges should become independent of LEA control. The intention was partly to make them free to respond to 'customers' (mainly employers).

Social reconstructionism

■ Social reconstructionism claims that education can be a force for positive social change, including (and perhaps especially) for creating an improved individual who is able critically to address prevailing social norms and help change them for the better.

■ It shares a change orientation with the enterprise ideology, but the nature of the desired change is very different and more radical.

■ It shares with the progressivist a preference for active, problem-solving pedagogy. The social reconstructivist favours a focus on subject disciplines, autonomous learning, but with strong guidance from the teacher, and a strong emphasis on emancipatory and critical projects, as well as on personal development over social and economic improvement.

This ideology is not found in government policy, but is evident among some educationalists. It is articulated in 'What the Radical Right Is Doing to Teacher Education: a Radical Left Response' (Hill, 1992), which argues that:

■ the teaching profession is being proletarianized by reducing the amount of training required and by replacing theoretically based courses with on-the-job training.

■ changes to teacher education mean that teachers will no longer come to the job with a concern for equal opportunities, multi-culturalism and antiracism, antisexism, discussion of issues of sexuality, or any sort of social justice. They will simply have subject knowledge and classroom skills.

■ the above factors plus increased managerialism, low pay, job intensification and increasing 'teaching from the book' mean that not only are teachers suffering, but the education system as a whole is becoming impoverished.

■ the possibility of critically addressing inequalities in society has almost disappeared.

Table 3.5 The linkages between political and educational ideologies

Political ideology	Educational ideology	Linkages
Social democracy	Progressivism	Emphasis on personal development and social co-operation
Neo-conservatism	Traditionalism	Emphasis on order, hierarchies and cultural transmission
Neo-liberalism	Enterprise	Emphasis on competitiveness in a market environment both individually and internationally

The enterprise–traditionalism paradox

Similarly, there was a paradoxical relationship between, on the one hand, Conservative government rhetoric stressing the need for education and training to equip 'Great Britain plc' to compete effectively in the global market and, on the other, the setting up of an old-fashioned national curriculum with a stress on traditional teaching methods. Such a curriculum is unlikely to enable Britain's workforce to compete in an international environment.

The idealistic rhetoric–pragmatic practice paradox

While government rhetoric stressed the need for training in high-level skills to be competitive internationally, in practice it is largely the low-attaining students who attend 'vocational' courses, which are usually oriented to the low-status, low-skilled, occupations. The reason behind this is that government had an urgent need to address the unemployment problem, and the unemployed were largely unable to benefit from training in higher-level skills.

However, it is not only New Right ideology which leads to paradoxes of policy like these. One example is:

The widening participation while increasing financial obstacles to learning paradox

Widening participation and enhancing lifelong learning have been two key themes in Labour post-compulsory education policy since 1997. However, while one set of policies has been designed to achieve this aim, largely employing changes to funding instruments for institutions, another set of policies has prevented them being successful. The abolition of maintenance grants for students and the introduction of contributions towards university fees, for example, led to a dramatic slowdown in the recruitment of mature students to universities in the late 1990s.

Key points

* The policy-making process is a complex one involving a contest between competing interpretations of 'the problem', negotiations and compromises during the policy-formulation stage.
* Between 1979 and 1997 there was a decline in the pluralistic nature of education policy formulation, with teachers' groups and LEAs especially progressively excluded, but with New Right think tanks increasingly drawn into the policy loop.
* Political and educational ideologies are important in the policy process. Understanding them helps the analyst to grasp underlying consistencies in values and attitudes and what the various players bring to the policy-making process. Table 3.6 provides a summary of some of the issues discussed in this respect. However, the linkages indicated in that table are loosely coupled ones. For example, the new Labour government of 1997 espoused a social democratic political ideology, yet some of its educational policies, such as its stress on the 3Rs and critique of project work (Bright 1997, p. 1), lay in the traditionalist ideological camp.
* Outcomes of the policy process are often unpredictable and contradictory, even when governments are strongly 'ideological', as those of the 1980s were. For example, despite the intention behind the national curriculum to lay greater stress on the 3Rs, the time available for these was squeezed in primary schools by a curriculum content over-full with other subjects.

Table 3.6 Ideological repertoires of education

Political ideology	Social democratic	Neo-liberal	Neo-conservative	Marxist, feminist and other conflict models
Educational ideology	Progressive	Enterprise	Traditionalist	Social reconstructionism
View of purpose of education	Personal and social development	Increase human capital	Socialization into norms and values of dominant culture	To empower marginalized groups and to change the status quo in the interests of equity
View of pupil or student	Entitlee	Raw material	Empty vessel	Change agent
View of parents	Partners	Supporters	Inadequate parents are a problem	Could be involved in pressing for change
View of teachers and other stakeholders	Partners	Some teachers too anti-business. Industry and commerce should be partners	Teachers can be too permissive. Other partners welcome if they accept educational philosophy.	Can represent an obstacle to change or facilitate it
Role of government	First among equal partners	Minimal	Retains control	Usually repressive
Appropriate curriculum	Student-centred	Vocational	Traditional	Developing critical thinking and linking theory and action

Source adapted from Dale 1989

Guide to further reading

On the role and power of the civil service within the DES, and generally for a discussion of pluralism and the changing role of government in education policy-making see:

Gewirtz, S. and Ozga, J. (1990) 'Partnership, pluralism and education policy: a reassessment', *Journal of Education Policy*, 5, pp. 37–48.

McPherson, A. and Raab, C. (1988) *Governing Education: A Sociology of Policy since 1945*, Edinburgh: Edinburgh University Press.

For more analysis of behind-the-scenes policy-making see:

Ball, S. J. (1990) *Politics and Policy Making in Education*, London: Routledge (especially Chapters 6 and 7).

Knight, C. (1990) *The Making of Tory Education Policy in Post-war Britain*, London: Falmer Press.

Lawton, D. (1994) *The Tory Mind on Education, 1979–94*, London: Falmer Press.

For some examples of the output of New Right think tanks see:

Ball, S. J. (1994) *Education Reform: A Critical and Post-structural Approach*, Buckingham: Open University Press, Chapter 3.

For more on political ideology see:

Gamble, A. (1988) *The Free Economy and the Strong State*, London: Macmillan.

Green, D. (ed.) (1991) *Empowering the Parents: How to Break the Schools' Monopoly*, London: Institute for Economic Affairs.

Hillgate Group (1987) *The Reform of British Education*, London: Hillgate Group.

Lawton, D. (1992) *Education and Politics in the 1990s: Conflict or Consensus?*, London: Falmer Press.

For an insight see:

Graham, Duncan (1993) *A Lesson For Us All? The Making of the National Curriculum* (with D. Tytler), London: Routledge.

A fascinating insider's account of policy-making on the national curriculum, a tell-it-like-it-was, step-by-step account from the inception to the first stages of implementation of the curriculum. The fact that Graham was forced to resign as a result of political manoeuvring makes him much more frank than most people in senior positions so soon after the events they descibe.

Useful websites

http://www.sosig.ac.uk
SOSIG (pronounced 'sausage') is the gateway to a number of extremely useful social science resources

http://www.staffs.ac.uk/journal/vol1no1/index.htm
The journal *Widening Participation and Lifelong Learning: The Journal of the Institute for Access Studies and the European Access Network* includes a paper by Maggie Woodrow exploring some of the policy paradoxes in Labour's 1997–2001 term. Woodrow's article is at: http://www.staffs.ac.uk/journal/vol1no1/ed-2.htm

http://www.cps.org.uk/
The Centre for Policy Studies, an independent centre-right think tank which develops and publishes public policy proposals and arranges seminars and lectures on topical policy issues, founded by Margaret Thatcher and Keith Joseph in 1974

http://www.iea.org.uk/
The Institute for Economic Affairs: another right-wing policy think tank

http://www.ieps.org.uk.cwc.net/hillcole.html
The Institute for Education Policy Studies: a left-wing education policy think tank

http://www.psi.org.uk/intro.htm
The Policy Studies Institute conducts 'research which will promote economic well-being and improve quality of life'

http://www.dfes.gov.uk/frontend/index.shtml
Department for Education and Skills

http://www.lsda.org.uk
The Learning and Skills Development Agency, 'a strategic national resource for the development of policy and practice in post-16 education and training'

Chapter 4
Reception and implementation of education policy

OUTLINE
It was suggested in Chapter 3 that policy sociology applies sociological analysis to the processes of policy formulation and implementation, and to the relationship between them; that chapter examined the formulation of policy. This chapter focuses on the implementation of policy, and the links between formulation and implementation. It begins by contrasting the managerial approach, which adopts a top-down approach to and understanding of policy implementation, and the phenomenological approach, which adopts a bottom-up approach to it. The case study illustrates and draws out important concepts and theoretical points.

Managerial approaches to policy implementation

The 'top-down' approach

> Leaders of the organization must have a clear vision of the desired end state of the entire system [and] a clear commitment to making significant personal investment in developing and building commitment [among staff] to an inspirational vision . . . All of this requires conscious and explicit planning and managing . . . It cannot be left to chance or good intentions.
>
> (Beckhard and Pritchard 1992, pp. 4 and 15)

Education policies are formulated in a variety of locales: in central government, in national bodies associated with government, in local authorities or in educational institutions. However, they are always *implemented* by individuals and groups within organizations: schools, colleges and universities. Therefore aspects of the study of management are relevant to understanding education policy, particularly what is usually called *Organizational Development* (OD), which focuses on change in organizations.

Within OD various positions have been proposed, one of which may be called the 'managerial' or 'top-down' approach to policy implementation. The quote from Beckhard and Pritchard above sums up the central notion of the managerial approach to putting policy into effect: that leaders at the top of organizations should set goals within the framework of broader policy and, by pulling the right levers, secure their staff's commitment to them. If this occurs it is assumed that, given sufficient available resources, policy can be successfully implemented by direction from above.

From the managerial perspective, it is important to make sure that managers know how to create the right conditions for successful implementation, how to 'make it happen'. Researchers in this tradition have tried to help by compiling lists of the necessary conditions for successful implementation. Table 4.1 gives a summary of some of the factors they have identified.

Cultural manipulation is central to this kind of approach. Managers are offered levers to shape the attitudes, values, expectations and behaviour of those involved within the organization, including teachers and academic staff. Such approaches have been variously termed 'culturalism' (Parker 2000) or 'the new leadership approach' (Bryman 1999).

> Much of the contemporary material emphasizes the need to produce *cultural change* rather than merely structural change (Beckhard and Pritchard 1992, for example). This involves committing the organisation to attitudinal readjustment . . . Institutional leaders are encouraged to 'lead by example' in order to commit others to their vision . . . *Our investigation has convinced us that strategic change is cultural change, and cultural change is related to institutional mission.*
>
> (Robertson 1994, pp. 314–5, emphasis mine)

Table 4.1 What managers should do to implement policy successfully – the 'top-down' approach

---

- creating and sustaining the commitment of those involved
- having clear and stable policy objectives
- ensuring that the policy innovation has priority over competing demands
- ensuring that there is a real expectation of solid outcomes inherent in policy, not just a symbolic one
- ensuring that the causal theory which underlies the policy reform is correct and adequate
- allocating sufficient financial resources
- creating, as far as possible, a stable environment within which policy is being implemented

---

Source   adapted from Cerych and Sabatier 1986

Change is carried through, for example, by:

- socialization into the organizational culture through the use of:
  - symbols and rituals (logos, mission statements, prize days, etc.)
  - improved communication strategies (in-house journals, informal conversations, managing the flow of stories about the organization)
  - careful recruitment of new staff
- staff development and persuasion
- coercion and the use of threats (demotion, sacking)
- rewards for conformity, such as bonus payments, free holidays, promotion.

Organizational development and functionalism

Underlying this approach in the top-down and some OD perspectives is a functionalist view of organizational cultures. Rooted in the anthropological study of 'simple' societies, this view sees successful organizations as having a single, strong culture which is shared and enacted by everyone in the organization and is essential to them in their struggle with the environment. Organizational culture is thought to give members a sense of meaning and identity which provide significance and context for them. In short, it 'defines their reality through their myths, rituals and procedures' (Barber 1984). The 'organizational saga' (Clark 1972) (the stories about the organization, its founder(s) and its history) is considered an important element in this; it acts as a means of uniting members in a shared vision of past, present and future. From the functionalist perspective organizational culture shapes behaviour and, if strong enough, can facilitate united action towards common and agreed goals, thus improving organizational effectiveness.

> Organisational culture induces purpose, commitment, and order, provides meaning and social cohesion and clarifies and explains behavioural expectations. Culture influences an organisation through the people within it.
>
> (Masland 1985, p. 158)

Organizations which have weak, or multiple and conflicting, cultures are ineffective and likely to fail. Thus the manager who wishes to see education policy successfully transferred into practice should work to build a strong, coherent culture in their school, college or university. Given clear policy goals, a strong culture, sufficient resources and an understanding of how to bring about change, the strong manager relatively easily ensures that policy is carried out as intended by the policy-makers.

Problems with the 'top-down' approach

Research into the implementation process demonstrated that, even if managers made sure that all of the factors in Table 4.1 were present, this would not be enough to ensure adoption. It became clear that they are merely necessary, not sufficient, for policy to be put into practice. This rethinking of the earlier work was most famously expressed in Barrett and Fudge's (1981) commentary on the top-down approach.

> Much of the existing literature tends to take a 'managerial' perspective: the problems of implementation are defined in terms of co-ordination, control or obtaining 'compliance' with policy. Such a policy-centred . . . view of the process . . . tends

to play down issues such as power relations, conflicting interests and value systems between individuals and agencies responsible for making policy and those responsible for taking action.

(Barrett and Fudge (eds) 1981)

The functionalist view of organizational culture in particular has received sustained criticism. Researchers have noted that:

- Cultures are *constructed* as well as *enacted*, that is, people do not simply act out the culture that they find in an organization: they change it too (Tierney 1987).
- Organizational cultures are multiple rather than unitary, at least in large organizations, and there are competing sets of values and of understandings at work in the interpretation of policy innovations. Each organization has a specific, and multiple, cultural configuration which is highly unstable (Alvesson 2002).
- Organizational cultures are highly complex, they contain many 'stages of action' including *front-of-stage* (the public arena of official statements, in-house journals and marketing literature), *back-stage* (where deals are done behind closed doors) and *under-the-stage* (where gossip is purveyed in quiet corners and over coffee) (Becher 1988).
- Managers' attempts to manipulate culture in the desire to implement policy exactly as formulated is unethical.

  If I view as essentially insulting an uninvited attempt to make me over into someone else's version of a better human being, should it be any less offensive to the hired hands?

  (Fitzgerald 1988, p. 13)

- Even if successful, the imposition of a single set of norms and values would undermine an educational organization. Organizations such as universities need independent critical thinkers and the ability to learn from mistakes rather than slavish obedience to the 'approved' way of thinking and doing things (Willmott 1993).

Phenomenological approaches to policy implementation

Researchers increasingly acknowledged the importance of the *phenomenology* of innovation. They showed that the earlier managerial approach had given too much attention to the goals of central actors, both government and managers of institutions. The values, attitudes and perceptions of those lower down, who were doing the donkey work of putting policy into practice, had been ignored. These people often use strategies which in effect *change* policy. They inevitably have discretion in order to cope with uncertainty; as a result policies tend to evolve through the interactions of a multiplicity of actors. Consequently policy becomes *refracted* as it is implemented, that is, it becomes distorted and less coherent as it is interpreted and put into practice by ground-level actors, such as teachers.

The postmodern viewpoint

Additionally, the postmodernist understanding of contemporary society began to stress the existence of different 'life-worlds', small communities within the larger society with their own understandings of the nature of reality and of how to 'go on' in life. Moreover, society itself, characterized as 'postmodern', was now seen as highly fluid, constructed and reconstructed on a continual basis. Older ideas of fixed structures conditioning behaviour and imposing regularity and predictability on social life were undermined by postmodern theory. This theoretical movement also had the effect of stressing the unpredictablity of human behaviour in policy implementation, and so the unpredictability of policy outcomes as against policy intentions.

The power of actors in the policy process

Researchers in this tradition, then, view policy implementation as being at least partly a 'bottom-up' process. As Saunders notes, elaborating on his concept of the 'implementation staircase':

> policy is expressed in a number of practices, e.g. the production of texts and rhetoric and the expression of project and national policy management, in school, in classrooms, and

in staffrooms. Policy is also expressed by different participants who exist in a matrix of differential, although not simply, hierarchic power. Finally, participants are both receivers and agents of policy and, as such, their 'production' of policy reflects priorities, pressures and interests characterising their location on an implementation staircase.

(Saunders 1986)

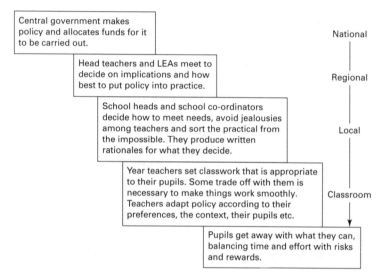

Figure 4.1 The implementation staircase

Source adapted from Saunders (1986) and Reynolds and Saunders (1987)

Policy, then, can be thought of as having a 'career', which begins at the point of formulation and progresses through the various stages of reception and implementation by the actors involved at different locations on the implementation staircase. A consequence of this is that researchers seeking to understand policy initiatives in their entirety should track them through each phase of their careers. Such studies are called *policy trajectory studies*, an example being Lingard and Garrick's 1997 study of the Social Justice Strategy in Queensland, Australia, discussed in more detail below.

The phenomenological perspective has come to be increasingly acknowledged in the study of education policy. In fact it underpins the whole subdiscipline of policy sociology. It stresses the importance of recognizing the role of implementation in actually *changing* policy. In a sense the implementation is actually part of the policy-making process itself, rather than being 'merely' a second stage of putting it into practice.

Another example of how policy is changed in its implementation comes from Michael Apple (1989), who tracks aspects of the proletarianization of school teachers in America, their de-skilling and the impoverishment of their working conditions. Yet he notes that:

> teachers have not stood by and accepted all this. . . . Militancy and political commitment are but one set of ways in which control is contested. It is also fought for on the job itself in subtle and even 'unconscious' (one might say 'cultural') ways.
>
> (Apple 1989, p. 48)

Similarly Michael Fullan's important and well-known work (1991; 1993; 1999) has shown the importance of school teachers' reactions in the implementation of education policies, drawing attention to the importance of the meaning of educational change (the title of one of his works) held by those on the ground (Fullan 1991).

Policy as text, policy as discourse

Policy as text

Stephen Ball (1994c), in discussing the issue of the power of local actors, distinguishes between policy as text and policy as discourse. This is a useful attempt to keep in view both the way behaviour and ideas are constrained by factors external to the individual (policy as discourse), and the relative freedom of individuals to change things (policy as text). The first is stressed by the 'top-down' approach, and the second by 'bottom-up' ones.

Viewing policy as text refers to the contested, changing and negotiated character of policy. Policy statements are always the outcome of struggle and compromise between the different individuals, groups and interests involved in policy-making. As Chapter 3 showed, the contested character of policy is evident at the initial stage of formal policy-making: the point of 'encoding' the ideas and values of the actors involved, as Ball puts it.

The disputed character of policy is also evident at the point of 'decoding' the text. Here individuals on the ground, such as teachers, interpret policy messages in the context of their own culture, ideology, history and resources. There is a close parallel with an audience watching and 'decoding' a television programme; the process is highly unpredictable and differs according to the characteristics of the audience viewing the programme (or policy) 'text'. In fact, researchers interested in audience reception of media texts have been engaged in the same sorts of debates about the power of media messages as education policy analysts have about the power of policy texts (see Trowler 1996, Chapter 2).

Ball sums up the idea of policy as text like this:

> [Once formulated,] policies shift and change their meaning in the arenas of politics; representations change, key interpreters . . . change . . . Policies are represented differently by different actors and interests.
>
> (Ball 1994c, pp. 16–17)

Policy as discourse

Regarding policy as *text* stresses the importance of social agency, of struggle and compromise, and the importance of understanding how policy is 'read'. This is balanced, however, by an understanding of *policy as discourse* (Ball 1994c; Bowe et al. 1994), in which the constraining effect of the discursive context set up by policy-makers comes to the fore. By discourse is meant the language or other forms of communication (e.g. pictures) that are used, the way ideas are expressed. Postmodernists such as Foucault emphasize the way in which the discourse available to us limits and shapes how we view the world. Ball draws on Foucault, who argues that discourses are:

> practices that systematically form the objects of which they speak . . . Discourses are not about objects; they do not identify objects, they constitute them and in the practice of doing so conceal their own invention.
>
> (Foucault 1977, p. 49)

Adapting the postmodern approach, Ball is here suggesting that discourse does not just represent reality, but helps to create it. Moreover, discourse 'disguises' the 'created' nature of social reality by denying the language resources needed to be able to think about and describe alternatives.

Policy-makers, then, can and do constrain the way we think about education in general, and specific education policies in particular, through the language in which they frame policies. Hargreaves and Reynolds (1989) illustrate this happening in schools in their discussion of the discourse in which national curriculum policy was presented. The notion that only 'core' and 'foundation' subjects need be addressed in the curriculum gave a solidity to those subjects and marginalized alternatives, such as development education, environmental education, political education. The latter are 'naturally' seen as peripheral, suitable only for less able groups. Meanwhile, it is quickly taken for granted that the core and foundation subjects are inherently superior.

What [was] contentious quickly become[s] normal, natural, reasonable, taken for granted. New subjects [are] eclipsed, forgotten, or consigned to older, less able groups. 'Real' subjects [are] distinguished from and thereby presented as self-evidently superior to mere 'clutter'.

(Hargreaves and Reynolds 1989, pp. 16–17)

Similarly Trowler (2001) shows how the discourse of New Higher Education in the UK frames the higher education system as a market catering to students as customers, situates knowledge as a commodity to be acquired and accumulated like any other and positions learning as involving the serial acquisition of learning outcomes, all available on the open market. The use of discursive repertoires drawn from business, marketing and finance is one of the ways by which this is accomplished: 'franchising', 'credit accumulation', 'delivery of learning outcomes', the 'possession' of skills and competences, skills 'audit' and the rest can become part of everyday discourse and begin to structure the way people think about education. Perhaps most importantly they work to exclude other possible ways of conceptualizing the nature of education. In this way they can begin to affect the practices which students, lecturers and others engage in, changing the nature of daily life in higher education and the assumptions and values found there. Trowler concludes, however, that this is not inevitable and that there is considerable scope for resistance and reconstruction of dominant discourses. Academic staff and students are not 'captured' by the discourse of New Higher Education, or at least not inevitably so.

For Ball, though, we are 'captured by the discourse', at least to some extent. This is where the real power of policy-makers and managers lies, rather than in less subtle attempts to shift the levers of cultural manipulation. Fairclough's (2000) reading of New Labour's 'new language' casts some doubt on this conclusion, however. His analysis of the discourse of the 'Third Way' (see page 151), for example, sees it as an ongoing process of representing the social world from a particular position through New Labour's documents, speeches, interviews, etc. Labour's Third Way is discursively presented as a policy direction which transcends the old divisions between right and left, one that seeks out and finds what works rather than one that is just acceptable to political factions. Through the analysis of texts Fairclough shows the multiple ways in which this idea is communicated. Yet this Third Way discourse is not all-powerful: the gap between New Labour rhetoric and the reality of its actions is the point at which discursive representations of reality can be contested:

> The politics of language, the politics of the gap between reality and rhetoric, is a fundamental part of politics, and it includes . . . various types of gap . . . between what people say and what they do, between action which is linguistic and action which takes other forms, between what people implicitly claim they are through their styles of performing and what other evidence suggest they really are. Political opposition to New Labour focuses on all these types of gap – setting, for instance, the discourse of 'partnership' against how New Labour actually governs, new welfare or pensions regulations against the experiences of claimants, or Blair's relaxed and inclusive style against evidence of 'control-freakery'.
>
> (Fairclough 2000: 155–6)

Criticisms of the bottom-up approach

In making the distinction between policy as text and policy as discourse, between action and structure, Ball addresses some of the criticisms made of early bottom-up or phenomenological studies, summarized by Marsh and Rhodes (1992).

- Bottom-up approaches overestimate the discretion of the lower level actors and fail to recognize sufficiently the constraints on their behaviour.
- They do not explain the sources of actors' definitions of the situation, perceptions of the their own interests, etc. In fact these may come, directly or indirectly, from above.
- The upper levels set the ground rules for negotiation: this is not recognized by these approaches.
- Bottom-up theorists are not really engaged in 'implementation analysis'. They do not focus on the implementation of policies, but on understanding actor interaction in a specific policy sector (Sabatier 1986, pp. 35–6).
- The criticisms of the top-down model are overstated. One criticism is that policy making at the top is characterized by multiple agendas and ambiguities which create room for interpretation and manoeuvre below. However, during the Thatcher period for example, policies tended to have very clear objectives.

Retaining the notion of policy as discourse ensures that researchers do not fall into such traps, most of which over-estimate the power of actors locally, as compared to structural factors.

Management implications of the phenomenological approach

Just as the top-down approach has clear implications for management action, the phenomenological approach can be used as a guide for managers. Its central message is that the pre-existing values and attitudes of an organization's staff need to be understood and addressed when considering change. Individuals and groups have deeply rooted values and attitudes, and these are reinforced by behaviours repeated daily. In educational organizations particularly, individuals draw on their ideas and values in order to think critically and deploy arguments in support of their point of view. Attempts to impose policy are likely to result in resistance, subversion, non-compliance and ultimately failure. The successful manager and leader is likely to be the one who understands his or her organization's cultural patterns, someone who knows their way around the cultural undergrowth:

> Knowing your way around . . . certainly depends on knowing that [propositional knowledge] and knowing how [procedural knowledge]. But it depends on much more as well – having a sense of orientation, recognising problems and opportunities, perceiving how things work together, possessing a feel for the structure and texture of a domain. It encompasses not just explicit but tacit knowledge, not just focal awareness but peripheral awareness, not just a sense of what's there but what's interesting and valuable. . . . Better than knowing that, knowing how or like names for knowledge, knowing your way around resonates with the notion of a learning environment.
>
> (Perkins, 1996, p. v)

The need for ownership of change

The alternative, as Senge (1992), Fullan (1993) and others point out, is to encourage the development of a shared vision, one that attracts broad commitment because it reflects the personal vision of those involved. Establishing this kind of ownership of change is difficult. Understanding is almost always fuzzy at first, and is clarified through experience of change. A sense of ownership of policy developments can quickly vanish, and needs to be sustained by hands-on experience, by experimentation and by adaptation of policies to local circumstances.

Stressing the importance of establishing a consensual vision for the future does not absolve senior management of the responsibility for goal setting. Over-centralization leads to over-control and resistance, but solutions which are too decentralized lead to anarchy and chaos. Many authors stress the importance of 'trialability' in introducing policy, and of initial small-scale experimentation, which is one of the strengths of the incrementalist approach. Yet, without support from above, this risks the danger of 'enclaving' (i.e. being restricted to a small group of enthusiastic innovators) and of change becoming stalled. Senior management needs to provide leadership, but any goals provided need to be limited, achievable and to provide room for local negotiation and accommodation. Change is more likely to be successful when there is consensus above and pressure below, a 'change sandwich', rather than when it simply flows from above.

Writers in this tradition stress that the top-down/bottom-up relationship needs to be one of dialogue, negotiation and learning from experience. They believe that dialogue is best conducted on the basis of mutual comprehension; for managers it is particularly important to understand the nature of the cultural characteristics of their institution. Indeed, gaining this understanding is the first piece of advice which Fullan gives to head teachers committed to building their school into a learning organization (Fullan and Hargreaves 1992). Conversely, the attention of those at ground level may need to be directed outwards, to the environment in which the organization is operating and the constraints and forces which are found there.

Policy implementation as evolution

Studying policy implementation in practice and reflecting on the implications for managers has, then, led researchers to move beyond the top-down/bottom-up polarity, and to focus instead on 'directed collegiality', the ideal policy-making/implementation approach. Top-down and bottom-up approaches are synthesized into a third perspective, one which Majone and Wildavsky refer to as implementation as evolution.

> At one extreme, we have the ideal type of the perfectly formed policy idea; it only requires execution, and the only problems are ones of control. At the other extreme, the policy idea is only an expression of basic principles and aspira- tions. . . . In between, where we live, is a set of more or less developed potentialities embedded in pieces of legislation,

court decisions and bureaucratic plans. This land of poten-
tiality we claim as the territory of implementation analysis.

(Majone and Wildavsky 1978, quoted in
Jordan 1982)

The implementation as evolution approach to implementation
analysis seems a sensible and moderate one. Its application is exem-
plified in the work of Hjern and Hull (1982) and Palumbo and
Calista (1990). Case studies of the implementation of actual
innovations, such as the Rand Change Agent Study (1974–8), have
confirmed that 'mutual adaptation' is a key to success: the adaptation of the innovation to fit the local setting and adaptations by
local users to fit the innovation (Hall 1995).

Case study: using grant-maintained school policy politically

Deem and Davies (1991) provide an insider account of the responses
of one secondary school, Stantonbury in Milton Keynes, in using
government policy on opting out to grant-maintained status (GMS;
see p. 198) to achieve its own goals, which were quite different to
those envisaged by the national policy-makers who formulated the
GMS policy. Rosemary Deem was a county councillor and Chair of
the school governors, and Michael Davies a co-Director of the school.
In their paper they recount the process of how the school coped with
a difficult environment in an innovative way.

The school had been set up in 1974 with egalitarian ideals, and
many aspects of its provision were 'student-centred'. In particular, it
rejected selectivism and attempted to achieve the integrative
comprehensive ideal, rejecting streaming and attempting to achieve
social mix and social tolerance. The LEA (Buckinghamshire), however, was a strongly conservative one which rapidly moved from
benign conservatism to right-wing interventionism during the 1980s.
There was considerable pressure for a grammar school system in
Milton Keynes, and a campaign was orchestrated by right-wing
pressure groups criticizing A level exam results in the city, linking
these to low-standard comprehensive education.

The response of Stantonbury school was to use the 1988 legislation to opt out of local authority control, not in order to become selective but as a way of retaining its educational ideals in a hostile environment. There was opposition from the Borough Council, from the Labour Party locally, and from LEA officers and members. Most parents, however, were supportive, particularly after the school campaigned for their vote for GMS. The school governors in particular were very supportive of the school's plan, despite the fact that this made it difficult for those who were councillors; both the Conservative Party and the Labour Party opposed the plan, and the Labour Party tried to expel those who supported the opt-out plan. The governors of the school 'became a single united group prepared to spend whole weekends as well as many evenings at school, writing leaflets, delivering them and holding animated discussions' (Deem and Davies 1991, p. 166).

The tenor of that campaign was that GMS would ensure continuity and stability at the school: the continuation of its egalitarian, comprehensive philosophy, now reinforced by the increased power and control that GMS would give to its head teachers and governors. 'Safeguard Local Democracy' and 'A Stable Future for All Our Students' were two slogans that were used. The campaign proved successful, with a majority of parents voting in favour of opting out. The school left the local authority on 1 September 1990.

After opting out the school was visited by Thames TV for a *This Week* programme, shown in December 1990. This was highly critical of the school's egalitarian climate and allegedly low educational standards.

> The main concern of the programme was seemingly to demonstrate that comprehensive schools like Stantonbury are full of progressive ideas about education and social adjustment but do not teach the basic skills properly.
>
> (Deem and Davies 1991, p. 168)

Subsequent press coverage was situated on the same ideological ground: what Ball (1990a, p. 31) calls the 'discourse of derision': 'Can't read, write or count . . . you must live in Milton Keynes' (*Today*). Even the 'quality' press accepted the agenda set by the *This Week* programme and oriented their pieces around the progressive schools' failure to transmit basic skills. Despite this critique, however, Stantonbury continued to stand by its principles, taking advantage of the new independence conferred by grant-maintained status.

Commentary

This case study raises a number of important issues for our understanding of policy implementation.

- The first is the power of local actors to negotiate and adapt centrally formulated policy.

> We contend that a small number of people can, in circumstances such as the ones outlined here, influence the direction of educational policy implementation, irrespective of the intentions of the legislators and politicians . . . We hope that this paper has demonstrated just how powerful human agency can be in subverting the intentions of others in the educational change process.
>
> (Deem and Davies 1991, p. 154, p. 170)

Here there is a stress on agency rather than structure, or in Ball's terms, on policy as text.

- Second, however, the media 'framing' of the issues involved nicely illustrate Ball's point about the constraints imposed by discursive repertoires. Stantonbury's position was being discursively 'fixed' in ways which made it difficult, but not impossible, to continue in the same mode.
- Third, the case study shows that the nature of change is conditioned by what Deem and Davies call a 'political' rather than a 'rational' model. The rational model is based on a top-down approach to policy-making and implementation: given that all the necessary conditions are in place, policy will be successful and there will be no 'implementation gap' between outcomes, as originally envisaged, and those which actually occur. The political model, by contrast, is located in a bottom-up perspective, and stresses the importance of conflict and negotiation, of alliances and emnities, and of competing definitions of the situation and goals. All of this is important territory for policy sociology.

- Fourth, and linked to this, is the variety of change agents involved. Many studies of change, such as Michael Fullan's numerous excellent works, stress the importance of teachers as change agents. This study illustrates that others, particularly school governors and parents, are also important actors in the change process.
- Fifth, it is noticeable that the unintended or latent consequences of policy can be at least as important as those intended by the policy-makers. As Chapter 1 showed, the policy of opting out to GMS was based on the idea of schools becoming independent, market-driven institutions free of LEA control. The neo-liberal ideology underpinning these ideas was a far cry from the progressive ideology of some of the key players in this case study. Stantonbury combined the opting-out policy, originally framed in an entirely different context, with an educational ideology which valued the comprehensive ideal in a way unforeseen by those in the policy loop. Such combinations and potential sets of events are probably unforeseeable in the main, but can have extremely important consequences.
- Finally, this study confirms Ball's point introduced in Chapter 3:

> Policy is . . . an 'economy of power', a set of technologies and practices which are realized and struggled over in local settings. Policy is both text and action, words and deeds, it is what is enacted as well as what is intended. Policies are always incomplete in so far as they relate to or map on to the 'wild profusion' of local practice. Policies are crude and simple. Practice is sophisticated, contingent, complex and unstable.
>
> (Ball 1994c, p. 10)

Case study: the Social Justice Strategy

Stephen Ball makes the point that one of the analytical consequences of a dual understanding of policy, as both text and as discourse, is to conduct what he calls *policy trajectory studies*. By this he means ones which trace the progress of policy from its formulation stage (where struggles, interpretations and compromises are mapped) through to the recipients of policy at the ground level (where interpretations and implementation strategies are similarly mapped). The policy trajectory research strategy holds out the prospect of a much fuller, more rounded, understanding of the processes and outcomes of educational policy-making and implementation, of the constraining effects of the environment as well as the power of actors. An example is given here in this case study.

Lingard and Garrick's study, conducted between 1994 and 1995, follows the development and implementation of Social Justice Strategy in Queensland, Australia. By researching both the formulation of the Strategy within Queensland's Department of Education and its implementation in a Brisbane secondary school, 'Brookridge State High School', they are able to trace the policy process through its various stages and identify the nature and sources of 'policy refraction'. This term refers to the distortion of policy which takes place as a result of the interaction of competing interests and sets of values. Policy becomes disjointed and less coherent as it goes through the 'encoding' and 'decoding' processes: it is refracted (Taylor et al. 1997, p. 119).

Queensland's government had been influenced by thirty-two years of Conservative governments and, since 1989, by New Right thinking within a Labor administration. This had led to a conservative policy culture within the State's Department of Education. By *policy culture* Lingard and Garrick mean 'the structures and policy goals, and dominant discourses and practices within public bureaucracies which frame the possibilities for policy' (Lingard and Garrick 1997, p. 2).

Within this unsympathetic environment the Social Justice Strategy was aimed at maximizing access, participation and outcomes for disadvantaged students, including girls, some minority ethnic groups and the 'gifted and talented'. The impetus for the Strategy had come from the Commonwealth level of government. Thus the push for this policy development was one external to the agency centrally concerned with its detailed formulation, Queensland's Education Department: 'equity concerns were largely funded by the Commonwealth, peripheral to its core business and bureaucratically buried in the bowels of the Department' (Lingard and Garrick 1997, p. 6).

Clearly too there was a tension between managerialism and concerns for social justice in schooling within the Labor governments at both the Commonwealth and State (Queensland) levels. Lingard and Garrick note that putting those committed to market liberal economic ideology in charge of social justice policies is like putting mice in charge of the cheese shop. As a result the notion of 'social justice' that was encoded into the Social Justice Strategy was 'distorted, reconstituted [and] reworked'. One of their respondents noted:

> social justice in Queensland is a poor third to efficiency and devolution, . . . because if it was important, if they felt it was something that really had to be done, they would do it. It would get a lot more response from the Department. They would be pushing it more, they would make sure they would have the money. Anything they really want to do, they do.
>
> (quoted Lingard and Garrick 1997, p. 11)

Though the dice were loaded against the Strategy from the beginning, the creation of an Equity Directorate with Queensland's Education Department and the appointment of a dynamic and nationally respected 'femocrat' as its director helped to put some dynamism behind this policy development. The importance of this to the policy process was recognized by participants, especially by those who had previously been frustrated by the policy culture in the Department:

> It just can't be underestimated [*sic*] how significant it is having the Equity Director on the Executive, both symbolically and materially. For example, there would hardly be a committee within this Department that would not have a representative from the Equity Directorate . . . I find it hard to summarise just what a huge improvement it is to get something moving.
>
> (quoted Lingard and Garrick 1997, p. 7)

The general aims of the Strategy were translated into twelve actions which schools and the Department of Education should take with expected outputs associated with each. Examples included a non-discriminatory language policy and the establishment of a database on access. The Strategy was distributed to all schools in September 1993 and Brookridge got three copies (for a staff of forty-five). Fewer than half of the teachers at Brookridge read it right through and those who did read it either because they agreed with its tenets or because they were considering applying for promotion (demonstration of a commitment to social justice was at that time a criterion of promotion).

During this period the teachers at the school had been bombarded with policy-related materials: 'you can't read it all and you can't internalise the whole thing . . . it gets filed – sometimes in the waste paper bin . . . Definitely, the volume of information you just can't take it all in' (teacher quoted in Lingard and Garrick 1997, p. 10).

As in the UK at the same period, teachers were being flooded with documents about a national curriculum, training reform, changes in assessment, etc. which came from the local, regional and national levels. The Social Justice Strategy was simply one more policy development being thrown at them. Teachers found the document too wordy, they had difficulty getting access to it and they considered it to be the responsibility of others, primarily the school principal, to implement it. Moreover they tended to interpret social justice in terms of 'fairness', stressing the need for 'fair competition'. Many argued that the Social Justice Strategy made no difference because they had always operated fairly towards all students.

There were though some practical developments which resulted from the Strategy:

- Two teachers were elected and trained as Sexual Harassment Referral Officers.
- Teachers formed a Special Needs and Social Justice Committee.
- They discussed or were 'inserviced' on the Sexual Harassment Referral Process and the new Behaviour Management Programme.
- Equity issues were incorporated into the School Development Plan.
- Beyond the school, Regional Assistant Co-ordinators (Social Justice) were appointed as well as a Regional Contact Officer, and regional workshops for teachers were organized.

However, all this meant increased intensification of teachers' work, and many of them were sceptical about the prospects for the Strategy's success: most had only minimal involvement with it and only two Brookridge teachers rated their interest in it as 'very high'; 10 to 15 per cent were explicitly against taking action to develop equity, believing it to be 'a lot of hogwash' and 'social engineering'.

Lingard and Garrick do not attempt to evaluate the achievements of the Strategy, which would anyway become apparent only in the longer term. It seems likely, however, that any achievements would not meet the aspirations the Equity Directorate had for it given the following factors.

First, much of the Strategy seemed tangential to the core concerns of the classroom teachers, particularly at a time when managerialism and efficiency were becoming the dominant concerns, as well as during a period of large curriculum, assessment and other pedagogic changes. Teachers were suffering from 'innovation fatigue'.

Second, there was hostility to the central policy machine, particularly at a time of reduced staffing, cuts to teacher release and to professional development as well as general job intensification.

Third, an important factor in what engagement teachers had with the strategy was the fact that a demonstrable commitment to social justice was a criterion of appointment and promotion. When this was abolished, an important incentive was removed. As Arnot et al. (1996) point out, this kind of requirement is important in the success of equality strategy outcomes. Its abolition also sent important signals to teachers about the significance of the Strategy, as did the resignation of the Director of Equity who had steered the Strategy's development.

Fourth, the Strategy had no clear implementation proposals incorporated into it. Policy-makers had not learned the important lessons that ground-level actors are important to the success of policy and that they need time, involvement in policy production, professional development and a material interest in its implementation. Simply sending the policy to schools is a long way from adequate for success in this respect. As Lingard and Garrick state: 'more energy is expended in the internal state micropolitics necessary to the production of a policy text than to its institutionalisation' (Lingard and Garrick 1997, p. 16).

Fifth, related to this, policy-makers tended to treat teachers as 'empty vessels', waiting to be filled with ideas and approaches emanating from Central Office' (p. 9). They are not.

Commentary

This study illustrates well the complexity and contested nature of the 'encoding' process during the policy formulation stage, with competing interests, values and ideas in a hostile environment working to achieve a 'settlement' around the Social Justice Strategy, but one which still left room for considerable interpretation about what the Strategy was about and how it should be implemented.

In addition it documents the considerable policy 'refraction' which occurred as policy was converted into practice at Brookridge State High School. It identifies too the local contextual factors which led to that refraction and conditioned the shape it took: the overwork of teachers, their attitudes towards the Strategy and its provenance and the competing discursive constructions of social justice.

The study also illustrates the mistakes that policy formulators often seem to make and repeat:

- They do not often take into account the need to support policy implementation, thinking that once the hard job of policy-making is done they can send out the finished documents and wait for results.
- They do not realize that the constant accumulation of educational policy leads to system overload.
- They develop an 'innovation bundle' and think of it as a single policy (in this case with the name Social Justice Strategy). In a bundle of loosely defined and loosely coupled innovations each strand is subject to competing interpretations and alternative viewpoints. Implementation in these circumstances becomes extremely complex.

Key points

- The concept of policy is more complex than originally set out in the basic definition given in Chapter 3. Policy must be viewed as something which is in a state of constant interpretation, negotiation and change in a number of sites. It should be viewed, too, as both text and discourse. Education policy, then, is multi-dimensional in character.

- The understanding of policy and its implementation needs to take account both of the constraints on behaviour and of the importance of individuals and of free will. To pick up a metaphor used by Ball in discussing his data collection with elite policy-makers (Ball 1994b, p. 118), we need to follow the paths of individuals as they move across the landscape, but we need to be aware of the nature of the landscape too.

- The language of 'implementation' and the 'implementation perspective' (viewed as the study of putting already formulated policy into practice) needs to be used carefully. Policy is almost always a compromise and can be read in a number of ways; the encoding process is a contested one, as is the decoding process. Policy is reinterpreted and changed as it is put into effect. Therefore the distinction between policy-making and policy-implementation is more blurred than the language of 'implementation' would suggest: 'A response [to policy] must . . . be put together, constructed in context, offset against other expectations. All this involves creative social action, not robotic reactivity' (Ball 1994c, p. 19).

- Ideology and culture play important roles in conditioning policy-making and policy implementation. While Chapter 1 showed how political ideology is important in education policy-making, this chapter has demonstrated the importance of educational ideology in policy implementation. Education managers' and teachers' attitudes towards educational issues have an important impact on the way they interpret policy and put it into effect. Accepted ways of thinking and behaving set the context into which new policy flows, and act as a filter in the policy-implementation process, shaping the interpretation and negotiation of policy.

- The most effective innovations involve mutual understanding and readiness to compromise (or mutual adaptation), by both those propagating the policy and those implementing it. For successful implementation, educational managers need to be aware of the cultural configuration within their organization and to consider likely responses to innovations.

Guide to further reading

For examples of implementation case studies see:

Bowe, R., Ball, S. J. with Gold, A. (1992) *Reforming Education and Changing Schools: Case studies in Policy Sociology*, London: Routledge.

Carter, D. S. G. and O'Neill, M. H. (eds) (1995) *Case Studies in Educational Change: An International Perspective*, London: Falmer Press.

Crawford, M., Kydd, L. and Parker, S. (eds) (1994) *Educational Management in Action*, Buckingham: Open University Press.

Woods, P. and Wenham, P. (1995) 'Politics and Pedagogy: A Case Study in Appropriation', *Journal of Education Policy*, 10, 2, pp. 119–41. (Gives a fascinating account of the production, reception, mediation and implementation of the 'Three Wise Men' report *Curriculum Organization and Classroom Practice in Primary Schools* (see p. 178).)

For managerialist approaches see:

Beckhard, R. and Pritchard, W. (1992) *Changing the Essence: The Art of Creating and Leading Fundamental Change in Organisations*, San Francisco: Jossey Bass.

For phenomenological approaches see:

Jermier, J. M., Knights, D. and Nord, W. R. (eds) (1994) *Resistance and Power in Organizations*, London: Routledge.

Lipsky, M. (1980) *Street Level Bureaucracy: Dilemmas of the Individual in Public Services*, Beverly Hills: Sage.

Robertson, D. (1994) *Choosing to Change*, London: HEQC.

For some good summaries of the field see:

Carter, D. S. G. and O'Neill, M. H. (eds) (1995) *Case Studies in Educational Change: International Perspectives on Educational Reform and Policy Implementation*, London: Falmer Press.

Ham, C. and Hill, M. (1993) *The Policy Process in the Modern Capitalist State*, Brighton: Wheatsheaf Books, 2nd edition.

Hill, M. (1993) *The Policy Process: A Reader*, Hemel Hempstead: Harvester Wheatsheaf. (A collection of some of the classic papers on policy, policy-making and policy implementation, though it follows the usual practice of policy studies of ignoring education in the main.)

Marsh, D. and Rhodes, R. A. W. (1992) *Implementing Thatcherite Policies*, Buckingham: The Society for Research into Higher Education and Open University Press.

Sabatier, P. (1986) 'Top-down and Bottom-up Approaches to Policy Implementation Research', *Journal of Public Policy*, 6, pp. 21–48.

Taylor, S., Rizvi, F., Lingard, B. and Henry, M. (1997) *Educational Policy and the Politics of Change*, London: Routledge.

For an insight see:

Chitty, Clyde and Simon, Brian (eds) (1993) *Education Answers Back: Critical Responses to Government Policy*, London: Lawrence and Wishart. This provides an extremely readable series of extracts from speeches and articles, written in the main by educationalists critical of government policy. These include Eric Bolton, head of Her Majesty's Inspectors until 1991, and several others who were once education insiders but became critical of the government's education policy. It thus gives an interesting insight into policy reception from a range of people in different locations, as well as interesting details from insiders on the actual impact of education policy as against the claims made for it. Particularly interesting and revealing are: Eric Bolton, 'Imaginary Gardens with Real Toads', Jim Campbell, 'The National Curriculum in Primary Schools: a Dream at Conception, a Nightmare at Delivery' and Sir Malcolm Thornton, 'The Role of the Government in Education'. Rather funny is John Patten's speech to the Conservative Party Conference in 1992 when he was education secretary ('I want William Shakespeare in our classrooms, not Ronald MacDonald'). Also included is John Major's famous 'Call me old fashioned' speech on education to the same conference.

Chapter 5
Government intervention in education

OUTLINE
This chapter sets out some of the key issues in education that governments have addressed or need to address. It also considers the legacy of eighteen years of Conservative administration prior to the Labour administrations of the late 1990s and early years of the twenty-first century. It then goes on to outline a number of pitfalls concerning education policy that governments have often fallen into in the past. Each of these represents a danger to the successful formulation and implementation of policies.

Labour inherits a Conservative legacy

Education will be our number one priority, and we will increase the share of national income spent on education as we decrease it on the bills of economic and social failure.

(Labour Party Manifesto 1997)

The New Labour strategy is to move forward where Margaret Thatcher left off.

(Mandelson and Liddle 1996, p. xx)

We have seen real improvements in the last four years. We have laid the foundations with increased investment, lower class sizes and rising primary school standards . . . Our education manifesto starts with a commitment further to increase the share of national income devoted to education . . . The challenge for us – and for our nation – in the next four years is to build on those foundations to see the investment and reform that our schools, colleges and universities all need.

(David Blunkett, Labour's Education Manifesto, 2001)

On its election in May 1997 the New Labour government promised that education would be its main priority: 'education, education, education' was the key to Britain's future, according to Tony Blair. A historical perspective might have dampened his optimism: in the 1960s American president Lyndon B. Johnson declared that 'the answer to all our national problems comes down to a single word: "education"', but this proved not to be the case.

The education system which the Labour government inherited had seen dramatic changes during the years of Conservative government, as Chapters 1 and 2 showed. There were some successes, but there were also numerous failures. In 1997 both higher and further education were suffering a crisis of funding after years of expansion in student numbers but relative reductions in funding. The unit of resource (funding per student) in FE was cut by around 28 per cent in further and higher education between 1992 and 1996 (Watson 1996; Thomson 1997). As a result, at least ten universities were on the financial 'sick list'; and the FE sector as a whole was £112 million in deficit with ninety-three 'sick' colleges. As the 1996 Dearing Report noted, a number of initiatives had been launched in schools and colleges at considerable expense but with only limited success. Examples included the national records of achievement initiative, a variety of schemes for youth training, and the nursery vouchers scheme. The new system of school inspections had caused much additional work, anxiety and expense in schools. Levels of truancy and permanent exclusions from school had increased dramatically during the early 1990s; exclusions, for example, rose from almost three thousand in 1990/1 to over eleven thousand in 1993/4 (*Guardian*, 26 June 1996). Some schools, such as the Ridings in Yorkshire, were failing spectacularly. Some blamed the marketization of the school system as a whole for this, arguing that it was creating a polarization of 'magnet' and 'sink' schools.

On the plus side, however, there were a number of successes. The Technical and Vocational Education Initiative (TVEI) was, by the end of its life, widely thought to have been a 'good thing', with many benefits for most students in the schools and colleges involved. The initial problems with the national curriculum were largely sorted out by the 1993 Dearing Report, and by 1997 it was operating reasonably well. Even the troublesome interface between Key Stage 4, tested at 16, and GCSEs was being smoothed out by 1997. Changes made to the inspection system had improved it, although problems remained. Meanwhile, most heads and governors, and many teachers, were enthusiastic about the benefits that local management of schools had brought, despite the obvious drawbacks (Marren and Levacic 1994). Labour retained much of the Conservative legacy, and in some cases was probably right to do so. In other cases, though, retention rather than change or abolition was largely a bad idea. Aspects of policy which survived the change of government relatively unscathed included the content of the national curriculum (the 'curriculum of the dead'); national tests; school league tables (albeit with a planned 'value added' element); the competitive school system; selectivism within schools; and the OFSTED model of inspection. In these cases there were convincing arguments for reform, at least.

The New Labour government itself claimed to be charting a 'third way' in its policy – a course which avoided the excesses of Conservative marketization on the one hand and central control of 'old Labour' policy on the other. Both the state regulation advocated by the old left and the deregulative, market-based approaches of the new right are rejected. With the Third Way policies are presented as being developed on the basis of 'what works', particularly when they are 'joined-up' policies: ones that reflect coherence across the different government departments' thinking. However, Power and Whitty (1999) conclude that:

First, in terms of the balance between old left and new right, there can be little doubt that the 'middle way' is skewed heavily to the new right ... It might be more accurate to suggest that New Labour's programme is based on a combination of 'what's popular' and 'what's easy' rather than 'what works'.

(Power and Whitty 1999, p. 541)

At the beginning of the twenty-first century there remain five key issues for education policy to tackle; they are dealt with below. In summary they are:

- improving educational provision
- tackling social disadvantage and improving equality of opportunity
- lifting the education profession
- improving the management of education
- shaping a learning society.

Five key issues in education policy

Improving educational provision

The raising of educational standards generally is a central plank of Labour government policies. The government has made clear its belief that some of the nation's schools have not so far helped children to achieve their full potential. In post-compulsory education the government is keen to maintain standards, and to support and extend centres of excellence. In fact 'excellence' is the key word throughout the education system and sums up the government's aspirations. The White Paper *Excellence in Schools* points out that:

- in the 1996 national tests only 60 per cent of 11 year olds reached the standard in maths and English expected for their age
- well over a third of 14 year olds were not achieving the level expected for their age in English, maths or science
- over 50 per cent of 16 year olds do not achieve five or more higher grade GCSEs, two-thirds of them do not achieve a grade C in maths and English, and one in twelve achieves no GCSEs at all
- international comparisons support the view that pupils in the UK are not achieving their potential; for example, 9 and 13 year olds were well down the rankings in the maths tests in the Third International Maths and Science Survey, the most recent international study
- OFSTED estimates that around 3 per cent of schools are failing, one in ten has a serious weakness in particular areas, and about a third are not as good as they should be.

The factors underlying this claimed failure to achieve potential are numerous and interrelated. Funding is clearly an important issue, and the Labour government in the early months of its first term of office made a series of funding announcements to improve resourcing in both compulsory and post-compulsory education. For New Labour other important factors were the need for a new partnership with all those involved in education, especially parents, and the need to reward successful teachers and schools, but to take action where there is failure. The introduction of new communication technologies in schools which would allow them to improve was also important for Labour policy. The four years between 1997 and 2001 saw a significant rise in SAT and GCSE results and, naturally, the government attributed these to the measures it had put in place.

Largely absent, however, was a recognition of and a determination to tackle the socio-economic causes of underachievement, located in structured class, ethnic and other patterned disadvantage. In this Labour had accepted the Conservatives' educational discourse of 'parents' and 'children' (e.g. '14 year olds'), which makes invisible the fractured nature of these categories and hides structured patterns of advantage and disadvantage, achievement and underachievement. This is evident in the way the problem is articulated in *Excellence in Schools*, as in the citation above; there is no mention of which categories of children are underachieving. Similarly, the policies on widening participation in post-compulsory education adopted an individualistic approach, failing to recognize the collective character of disadvantage and the socio-economic roots of low participation levels among some groups. This leads to the next point.

Tackling social disadvantage and improving equality of opportunity

Patterns of disadvantage

It is clear that there are a number of gaps in educational opportunity that need to be addressed by any government for which this is a concern.

First there is the issue of general patterns of underachievement by some groups.

- Boys generally tend to do badly in English and maths compared to girls at the ages of 7 and 14 (SATs at Key Stages 1 and 3) (Gipps and Murphy 1994).
- In general boys do worse than girls at public examinations (GCSE and GCE A levels).
- Men are more likely than women to achieve first-class degrees, though they are also more likely to fail and get third-class degrees.
- Some minority ethnic groups do badly in public examinations compared to others, particularly Bangladeshis and Pakistanis. Others, e.g. Africans, do well.
- Afro-Caribbean pupils tend not to achieve higher grades of pass in public examinations as frequently as some other groups.
- Schools with largely middle-class intakes have better public examination and SAT results than those with largely working-class intakes.

Second is the question of access to the whole curriculum and to post-compulsory education.

- Afro-Caribbean students constituted 56 per cent of all permanent exclusions in one local authority studied (Gewirtz et al. 1995). This is disturbing given the rapid increase in the number of permanent exclusions in the early 1990s.
- People from ethnic minorities are more likely to continue into post-compulsory education than the 'white' population; but for some it is more likely to be men that stay on, while in others it is more often women (Labour Force Surveys). Many minority ethnic groups are also better represented than the 'white' population in higher education (Modood 1993), as well as in further education and training schemes.
- Students with fathers in non-manual occupations are more likely to go to university, the chances increasing with the higher socio-economic status of the father (OPCS 1989).
- The higher the social class of a student's father, the greater is the

likelihood of that student attending a high-status course (e.g. law or medicine) at university.

- In post-compulsory education there remains a clear distinction between subjects predominantly studied by men and those 'chosen' by women. This has important implications for subsequent careers, and levels of pay and status. The same applies where choice is permitted in schools.
- Only around 3 per cent of the university population define themselves as having special needs, considerably less than in the population at large.

Coherence in policies to tackle disadvantage

Labour is concerned to raise the standards but tends to lack coherence in its policies designed to reduce differentials such as these: 'To those who say where is Labour's passion for social justice, I say education is social justice' (Tony Blair, *Times Educational Supplement*, 18 April 1997). The early focus of the government elected in 1997 was on raising standards for all: a laudable aim, but one that makes patterns of privilege and disadvantage invisible. Later policies, especially the *Excellence in Cities* initiative, did move to focus resources and policy on the disadvantaged, yet others (for example those concerned with widening participation in higher education) lacked an equally targeted approach and were individualistic rather than collective in their approach to the problem. Labour continues to be concerned with developing an inclusive society, in which everyone gains from prosperity, and not, for example, equality in outcomes. Thus there is no attempt to tackle the privilege for some provided by the private education sector. The Education Action Zones initiative released relatively limited additional resources for city schools, with a failure to attract adequate private funding into the venture. The effects of the targeted resources were likewise small. Certainly the history of similar initiatives in the past, such as the Education Priority Areas and Community Development Programmes in the 1970s, suggest that the prospects of their improving equity in education are not good (Hayter 1997). Nor does the government appear to understand, or have policies to tackle, the patterned nature of educational

advantage and disadvantage structured by different levels of possession of 'cultural capital', the resources available to some which
advantage them in all aspects of education from admission to exit.
These gaps in education policy are most evident in Labour's
policy on selectivism. In the final years of the Thatcher government
selectivism was on the increase within the state school system. Early
limits on the degree of selection which schools could impose were
quickly lifted, so that 15 per cent of the entry could be admitted
after a test of ability. Proposals quickly followed to allow 20 per cent
of the intake of comprehensives to be selected by ability, 30 per cent
for city technology colleges and 50 per cent for grant-maintained
schools. Internally, selectivism by ability was encouraged, with
streaming or banding of year groups across the school and setting
by subject becoming the norm. This continues with the *Excellence
in Cities'* stress on setting within secondary schools.

Labour has not mounted an attack against selectivism by schools
or within their walls. On the contrary, the government favours
selectivism both for entry to schools and within them. Grant-
maintained schools will become 'foundation schools', and will
undoubtedly continue to be perceived as more desirable by parents
than LEA-controlled community schools. Grammar schools, wherever they exist, will almost certainly remain. Given that Labour will
allow parents to decide their future, it is highly unlikely they
will vote for comprehensivization. New specialist schools are to
be encouraged, selecting pupils by aptitude.

Within schools, selectivism (streaming, setting, banding or within-
class grouping) is to be the norm. 'Diversity within one campus' is
the catch phrase which the government uses, justifying its stress
on selectivism within schools on the grounds that mixed-ability
teaching is effective only when done by highly skilled teachers, and
that usually it does not bring out the potential abilities of most
children.

The problem with this is that the weight of research evidence
shows that selectivism by and within schools operates against the
already disadvantaged in education and in favour of those who
already have advantage. A review of the available literature on
the subject conducted by Harlen and Malcolm (1997) found no
consistent and reliable evidence of positive effects of setting and

streaming in any subjects or for students of particular ability levels. The disadvantages of setting or streaming are well known, however: social class and other divisions are reinforced, there is an increased likelihood of delinquent behaviour in the later years of schooling, and teacher expectations are lowered for those defined as less able.

Lifting the education profession

During the 1980s the education profession came under serious attack from the government. Ball (1990a) talks about the 'discourse of derision', referring to the way in which teaching was consistently portrayed as an incompetent, politically motivated, self-interested profession, unthinkingly attached to progressivist dogmas of teaching peddled by university teacher-training departments. Those on the left (e.g. Hill 1992) saw this as part of a social engineering agenda: an attempt to mute those who wished to see education developing critical faculties in children.

Changes to the education profession were interpreted in these terms. The move away from theoretically based teacher education in universities towards classroom-based training was seen as a move to turn teachers into technicians with skills, rather than independent and reflective professionals with a strong theoretical base to their actions. The introduction of teacher qualification programmes with very little preparation prior to classroom experience, such as the licensed teacher and articled teacher schemes, were aspects of the same agenda from this point of view.

Meanwhile, the development of the national curriculum and the associated teaching and testing materials led to a separation of conception from execution (Apple 1989), with the thinking and planning increasingly being done by curriculum designers and textbook authors, and teachers merely 'delivering' a product. As well as having a political agenda, such developments were interpreted as aspects of Fordism: the application of production-line methods to education with a consequent de-skilling of teachers, who are now required to perform repetitive unskilled tasks.

In further and higher education there were clear signs of post-Fordist patterns (Carter 1997). Professionals were increasingly employed on temporary or part-time contracts, often not renewed.

The core of permanent professionals shrank while the periphery of 'flexible' workers, often poorly paid, grew dramatically in the late 1980s and 1990s. For some writers (e.g. Ball 1990a) these developments were explained in terms of a response to a financial crisis in capitalism. Whatever the causes, it was clear that the combination of Fordist and post-Fordist developments as well as a general decline in resourcing for education had, by the mid-1990s, led to the following for a significant proportion of educational professionals across the sectors:

- work degradation: a decline in the conditions at work, the materials available, the physical surroundings, the environment
- work intensification: an increase in the amount that was expected to be done with a corresponding decline in the resources available to do it: in short, more for less
- de-skilling: a decline in the level of skill required to do the job and a consequent decline in professional standing: a move towards technician status; this is increasingly reflected in changes in job titles and levels of pay, particularly in the further education sector, as well as in changes to teacher education
- bureaucratization: the increasing requirement to complete paperwork, provide information, complete records, all of which compound the processes of work intensification and de-skilling
- work 'flexibility': an increase in job contracts which are short-term and part-time, with central agencies providing teachers and lecturers for specific purposes
- loss of control over the work process and hence loss of job satisfaction
- reduced control over the use of time as managerialist practices increasingly controlling what teachers do and when they do it.

The effectiveness of the proposed General Teaching Council in acting as a voice for the education profession in the face of such pressures will almost certainly be hampered by the continuing existence of the Teacher Training Agency. The TTA has taken numerous powers to itself in the short period it has been in existence, powers which in Scotland belong to the Scottish equivalent of the General Teaching Council. Clearly, there will be pressure from the TTA to retain those powers; this is likely both to weaken the GTC south of the border and to create tensions between the two organizations.

Kogan points out that this kind of issue is particularly important in contemporary educational change, which tends to be:

> negotiated through conflicts between and within bureaucratic, economic and social demands. In an increasingly complex society group interests and the ideologies supporting them are experienced chiefly through highly bureaucratised institutions which establish their own logic of development. But nothing is automatic. Changes occur, sometimes accidentally, when the right configuration of feelings, ideologies and power coincide.
>
> (Kogan 1982, p. 6, quoted in Ball 1990a, p. 16)

Labour's discourse, and that of much educational research, appears to centre on 'good' and 'bad' teachers; the former to be lauded and the latter to be chastised, even named and shamed. In this they appear to be adopting, albeit in a more muted form, the 'discourse of derision' which has undermined teachers' status, self-confidence and credibility. Such a policy cannot lead to improvements in the education service.

Improving the management of education

During the 1980s a process of restructuring went on in educational management. This involved a changing emphasis in a number of areas. There was a move to the measurement and improvement of the outputs of education, particularly examination results, rather than on the processes of schooling. Performance indicators, such as the number of A level passes, the post-16 staying-on rate, levels of truancy and SAT scores, became the key to evaluating the performance of schools and so became a prime concern of education managers. Higher standards became defined in these terms, and there was a shift of concern away from the development of the individual and the quality of the educational process itself. The establishment of a set of national training targets was mirrored by similar local sets of quantitative targets. The question became not: 'Is what we are doing the right thing and are we doing it well?' Rather it was: 'How efficient and effective are we at achieving the goals that have been set for us?' Educational management became largely viewed as applying a set of tools, derived from management approaches in other contexts, to the task that had been set. The training of school and college managers likewise became seen in terms of enhancing their understanding of these tools and their ability to use them: the development of a set of skills. The National College for School Leadership, set up in 2000, looks set to continue this approach. It advocates the compentency-based approach which sees good leadership as inhering in the personal characteristics demonstrated by individual leaders and sees its task in terms of enhancing desirable personal characteristics. Meanwhile ideas and practices based on management in industry began to pervade schools and other institutions, and the discourse of educational management began to change. Head teachers and their colleagues became 'line managers' and 'directors', performance objectives were prescribed for teachers at appraisal interviews, charters and service standards for 'customers' and 'clients' were developed. Gewirtz et al. (1995) sum up some of the these changes in Table 5.1.

While this new managerialist ethos has brought some improvements to the quality of educational provision, it has also brought a new set of ideas and practices to the education service, many of which are inappropriate to it. Education management involves more than the attempt to achieve a set of imposed quantitative goals as efficiently as possible. Good managers and leaders are involved in formulating and evaluating goals, and they involve their colleagues in that task. They understand the staff and students in their institution and are able to work with them. They are thinking, reflective practitioners, not merely the skilled users of a set of generic management tools.

Although previous governments have rightly identified the development of education management as a key issue for school and college improvement, they have to date gone about it in the wrong way. To date the Labour government has accepted the structures, approach and discourse of previous governments which, on the whole, have been antipathetic to the education profession.

Table 5.1 The shift from bureau-professionalism to new managerialism

Bureau-professionalism	New managerialism
Public service ethos	Customer-oriented ethos
Decisions driven by commitment to 'professional standards' and values, e.g. equity, care and social justice	Decisions driven by efficiency, cost-effectiveness and search for competitive edge
Emphasis on collective relations with employees through trade unions	Emphasis on individual relations through marginalization of trade unions, and new management techniques
Consultative	Macho
Emphasis on the educative process and on the quality of interaction between teacher and learners, learners and learners	Emphasis on efficiency and effectiveness, the achievement of planned outcomes
Co-operation	Competition
Managers socialized within field and values of education sector	Managers trained in generic field of management

Source adapted from Gewirtz et al. (1995), p. 94

Shaping a learning society

The idea of a 'learning society' is one that emerges from a number of educational reports as being of central importance for the future of Britain and its education system (National Commission on Education 1993, 1995b; Dearing 1997). It is also an idea that is attracting much research attention owing to substantial funding from the Economic and Social Research Council for research into 'the learning society'. The phrase is intended to sum up a 'preferred future': a form of society which it is thought desirable to begin shaping now. Drawing from a number of sources, it is possible to say that the main features of a learning society comprise the following.

- Individuals, communities and organizations, as a matter of course, reflect on and learn from experience, and alter their

behaviour, ideas and purposes in appropriate ways as a result. This process happens with the benefit of the required knowledge and clarity of thought.
- Education and training are available to individuals throughout their lives at work, at home, in the community and in educational organizations, enabling them to achieve their potential.
- Individuals empowered by knowledge, skills and understanding can contribute fully and continuously at work and in the community.
- The benefits of a learning society include stronger communities, more effective businesses, greater international competitiveness, a richer culture and a more cohesive society.

What needs to be done? Again, drawing from a number of reports, it is possible to identify the following steps which most or all agree on.

- Conduct education policy-making in all education sectors with the underlying strategic aim of achieving the learning society.
- Improve the quality of learning, teaching and management in schools and colleges, and give teachers and educational managers status and ownership again.
- Ensure that students at whatever level are encouraged to perform beyond their own expectations: standards need to be set high.
- Be prepared to innovate in the educational field.
- Improve the provision and quality of early-years education.
- Improve the job prospects of low-achieving school-leavers.
- Undertake world-quality research and disseminate its results to the nation.
- Ensure that lack of resources is not a barrier to continuing education.

A good start has been made towards the achievement of a learning society. The government is committed to funding nursery places, there is a commitment to lifelong learning (a Green Paper was published in March 1998) and there is a commitment to raising the quality of teaching and learning, and to introducing (and funding) information and communication technology in all schools. Generally the resources allocated to education have increased substantially under the New Labour regime. Further steps were taken in 1997–2001. School-leaver training received the attention it badly needed and the rather disparate funding arrangements for further education were unified. In the second half of its period of office that government stopped tinkering with the system it inherited and began to make more fundamental changes in a series of bold initiatives. However, the lifelong learning policy thrust is based on an individualistic, market-oriented perspective. Occluded in such a perspective is the structured nature of exclusion from continuing education. Groups of people, not individuals, find participation difficult for important socio-economic reasons. Tackling the problem at the level of the individual 'consumer' of education is unlikely to solve it. Also marginalized in current policy is the notion of learning for other purposes than narrowly vocational ones. The danger in this is learning which prepares people for last year's tasks, not next year's, and at a more general level bringing about a Philistine society.

From a postmodernist perspective, the need for change in the education system is even more pressing and the required change even more dramatic. As Britain moves closer to the condition usually described as 'postmodernity', the education system becomes increasingly anachronistic. The global, dynamic, individualistic and playful nature of postmodern society is at odds with the staid authoritarianism of the school sector in particular. Moves towards the right-hand side of the table have been made in post-compulsory education, most notably in the shape of LearnDirect (see page 66). Table 5.2 summarizes some of the issues raised by this perspective on a learning society.

Four lessons for New Labour

Governments are not much inclined to pay heed to what educational researchers have to tell them, as the next chapter shows. This is a pity, for there is much that governments could learn from academic research both about the detail of education policy and about its implementation. Below are set out four clear lessons that Labour could learn from work that has been done by policy sociologists and others about education policy. In summary they are:

- Education can't fix everything: don't expect it to.
- Policy implementation is tough.
- Expect different outcomes in different contexts. Continue to devolve but provide direction.
- Be aware of the uses and limits of ideology.

Table 5.2 Postmodernity and education

Current education system (modernist)	Contradictions in a postmodern society	More appropriate education system
Dull, fixed content of national curriculum	Contrast with choices available through media and popular culture	Choice, interactivity, learner navigation
Knowledge clearly divided into high and low status	Mixing of 'high' and 'low' culture, standards of judgement open to question	Edutainment, educational games, presentation of material through multimedia
Hierarchical relationship in schools – authority expected to be unquestioned	Breakdown and questioning of authority, 'crisis of legitimation'	Individual responsibility for learning, perhaps with selected others
Regulation of behaviour through timetables, etc.	Postmodernity = the consumer society	Place and time of learning determined by the consumer of knowledge
Fixed curriculum and syllabuses	Rapid change in knowledge – 'future shock'	Knowledge 'consumed' as needed – 'just in time' education

Education can't fix everything: don't expect it to

Like previous governments, Labour initially underestimated the power of social structures, social divisions and disadvantage, while overestimating the power of education to overcome these. The idea of 'zero tolerance of under-performance', set out in the *Excellence in Schools* White Paper, makes little allowance for those schools with catchment areas in heavily deprived areas. Though the White Paper admits that problems of low standards and underperformance in some schools 'have deep roots', the expectation was that they could be solved through improving teachers and improving schools. Later in its term it began to recognize the scale of the problem: the *Excellence in Cities* initiative sought to address the weaknesses of the Education Action Zones set up early in the administration and to target funds where they were most needed. We have yet to see whether this has gone far enough. Later still, though, the notion of 'lifelong learning' was seen as 'a wonder drug which, on its own, will solve a wide range of educational, social and political ills' (Coffield 1999, p. 479).

In 1970 Basil Bernstein baldly stated that 'education cannot compensate for society'. What he meant by this was that social inequalities were so intractable that the education system as a whole does not exercise a powerful enough influence to mitigate the effects of social disadvantage.

More recently a review of the evidence on how far effective schools can compensate for society was conducted by Peter Mortimore, one of the leading researchers on effective schools (Mortimore 1997). He concluded that the best, most effective, individual schools can compensate for society to a certain extent, supporting individuals in their efforts to overcome the negative effects of social disadvantage. However, the success of such schools will be partial and limited, because those who are advantaged will tend to benefit more from any improvement in schools; so that, while all benefit from school improvement which derives from government and other policies, the advantaged benefit most.

For Mortimore the answer lies in a fair distribution of educational spending with, in some cases, additional spending directed towards schools which serve the most disadvantaged groups. However, critics of the school effectiveness or school improvement movement point out that the emphasis on the school detracts attention from the underlying social disadvantages: 'the school is to take responsibility for its ailments and its own cure' (Ball 1990a, p. 90). The emphasis on helping schools accepts uncritically the New Right model of schools as autonomous agencies. For critical theorists and others, tackling underachievement in schools is to tackle the symptom, not the disease. Socio-economic inequalities, racism and other forms of disadvantage are the priorities. Education cannot compensate for society.

Like most governments, Labour appears to believe that educating the population can solve many of the nation's social and economic problems, ranging from the excessive number of unwanted births to single mothers, criminal behaviour and welfare dependency, to a lack of international economic competitiveness. 'Britain's economic prosperity and social cohesion . . . depend on [creating] . . . a society in which everyone is well-educated and able to learn throughout life' (DfEE 1997, *Excellence in Schools*, p. 1).

Clark Kerr (1991) reviewed a range of evidence on the idea that education is the key to a nation's international competitiveness. He concluded that probably in no other area of policy-making have so many firm convictions held by so many been based on so little proof. A good education system is one, but only one, prerequisite for a successful economy and a more equitable society. Other inputs are required, and in their absence education is unlikely to be able to achieve the goals set for it by policy-makers. Some of the other inputs required to bring this about include:

- more employment opportunities for more productive workers
- new investment to take advantage of more productive approaches and new technologies
- new methods of work organization which take advantage of the increased productive capacity of better educated workers (e.g. ones that enable workers to exercise discretion in decision-making)
- new managerial approaches which support worker participation and create more integrated approaches to research, training, product development, marketing, production and finance (Levin and Kelley 1997)
- building motivation into policies so that, for example, employers are encouraged by incentives and sanctions to take equal opportunities seriously.

Peter Robinson in a study of education and economic performance (Robinson 1997) calculates that only 37 per cent of jobs require literacy to GCSE grade C and above, and 50 per cent of pupils already attain this level. It will take forty years before demand meets the supply, even assuming that the pass rate at GCSE stays level. Education, therefore, may not be the central factor in improving Britain's economic performance.

Policy implementation is tough

Chapter 4 explored how policy is reinterpreted and changed as it is put into effect. Policy-makers often forget that implementation of policy is at least as important as policy formulation. They consequently forget to plan for and adequately resource implementation. As Raab (1994, p. 24) puts it: 'the pudding eaten is a far cry from the original recipe'. To avoid this there are a number of requirements that need to be in place.

- There is a tremendous need to have a clear and deep understanding of exactly what the policy is intended to bring about. The nature of the innovation should be spelled out in very clear terms (Hall 1995, p. 112).
- Conditions that are supportive of implementation need to be created and sustained. These include:
  - resources
  - sufficient time for innovations to permeate
  - support and training for the professionals facilitating change.
- Clear guidance from above is needed, but room must be left for local interpretation and adjustment to policy.
- Policies need to be developed, and their implementation planned, with an understanding of the micropolitics that exist within change contexts. This will increase the chances of successful implementation at the ground level.
- Similarly the pre-existing values, attitudes, norms and understandings of those at the ground level need to be appreciated in order to predict and take into account the potential trajectory of policy as it moves from formulation to implementation.

The government's plans for a national grid for learning (NGfL) present an interesting case study of these issues. Its document

Connecting the Learning Society: National Grid for Learning (1997) appears to show awareness of the level of resourcing required, and a commitment to provide it. There is also a keen awareness of teachers' current lack of understanding of and confidence with information and communication technology, and hence the need for staff development in the area. What is lacking in the document is:

- an understanding of how teachers' attitudes towards the role of ICT in teaching and learning may lead to outcomes other than those intended (many will not see it as desirable or appropriate, for example)
- an understanding of how pupils and students will (mis)use the technology
- a clear understanding of precisely what it will be used for and how this will be an improvement over alternative uses of the resources.

Simply providing the infrastructure will not bring about desired outcomes, particularly if those outcomes are unclear to policy-makers and participants in the first place. Selwyn and Fitz (2001) have shown how the NGfL initiative stemmed from a very small elite group in the government, including the Prime Minister Tony Blair. There was a closely co-ordinated network involving the government and civil service in conceptualizing, formulating and steering the initiative. There was already in place a well-formed and stable network of public and private organizations and actors which had formed the basis of the educational ICT community two decades before the NGfL initiative. Yet despite this strong top-down direction and the stable basis for policy implementation Selwyn and Fitz's case-study research concludes that

> the compatibility of the NGfL with schools' objectives remains to be seen. As yet schools' reaction to the NGfL is unclear above and beyond the initial spending of government and lottery money. Whether the NGfL can be successful in creating a culture of ICT throughout the *whole* school sector is debatable . . . One foreseeable consequence of the Grid, therefore, is merely an exaggerated version of the pre-1997

education ICT picture; with some schools as technologically rich as others are equally as poor.

(Selwyn and Fitz, 2001, p 145)

Expect different outcomes in different contexts. Continue to devolve but provide direction

It is a clear finding from numerous studies of the impact of education policy in different locales that outcomes are rarely the same in different places. Studies by Woods et al. (1996), Gewirtz et al. (1995) and Arnot et al. (1996) on different aspects of education policy all conclude that outcomes are heavily dependent on local circumstances. In their study of equal opportunity of education policies during the Thatcher years, Arnot et al. reveal a very variable pattern, with equality of opportunity for males and females being advanced in some areas as a result of some policies, yet undermined in others. Woods' study of the impact of 'parental choice' policies on schools' behaviour shows that this very much depends on local circumstances, a finding confirmed by Gewirtz et al.'s broader study. Figure 5.1 illustrates some of the factors which condition local policy outcomes in this area. Gewirtz et al. conclude that:

there is no one general market in operation in England. Education markets are localised and need to be analysed and understood in terms of a set of complex dynamics which mediate and contextualise the impact and effects of the Government's policy.

(Gewirtz et al. 1995, p. 3)

Clearly, then, governments need to ensure that, while they set the direction of education policy, there is sufficient power at the local level to adapt it to local circumstances. Local education authorities, governors, head teachers and teachers are best placed to predict, evaluate and interpret the outcomes of policy, and to shape it appropriately for the circumstances they have to deal with.

Moreover, as Ball (1999) points out, the danger of central direction in education, through the numeracy hour and literacy

Education Policy

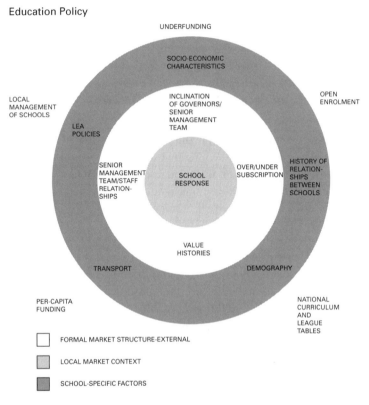

Figure 5.1 The impact of context on outcomes

Source adapted from Gewirtz et al. (1995) p. 88

hour, national curriculum schemes of work and the rest, is that *learning* is forgotten. School pupils are taught to pass tests and to follow centrally prescribed schemes of work, but they are not encouraged to process or apply this knowledge. Lauder et al. (1998) agree:

> the critical issue must surely be in part a question not only of text results but how they are arrived at . . . In England the problem of how to raise basic educational standards while preserving or developing creativity is not even part of the public debate . . . if we are not careful policy settings which

emphasise results at the expense of methods will lead to a trained incapacity to think openly and critically about problems that wil confront us in ten or twenty years' time throughout the system.

(Lauder et al. 1998, p. 15)

Be aware of the uses and limits of ideology

New Labour presents itself as free of the ideological thinking about education which pervaded policy-making in the past. Indeed, the 'new' in New Labour is primarily there as a marker to distinguish it from 'old' Labour, characterized (or caricatured) as blinkered by class-based thinking. Naturally, New Labour distinguishes itself from Margaret Thatcher's ideologically laden years in power, and the mistakes which were made as a result of similarly blinkered thinking. Instead the image presented is one of a practical orientation underpinned by a pluralist viewpoint: New Labour as the honest broker which listens to competing voices and makes sensible decisions based on sound common sense.

Certainly ideology does place limits on thinking. It defines what the important questions are, where the priorities lie, how issues should be viewed, and indicates the sorts of actions that can and should be taken. In the past, thinking in ideological terms has meant, for example, the exclusion of important actors on the education scene from participation in policy and decision-making. It has led to a lack of awareness of and an unwillingness to appreciate where policies were not working or were fundamentally misguided, as was the case with youth training policy and nursery vouchers. It has also led to limited thinking about the likely unwanted effects of policy, such as the consequences of 'parental choice' of schools, publication of examination statistics and so on for pupils with special needs or for schools in deprived catchment areas. Avoiding such detrimental effects of ideological thinking can only be for the good.

However, ideological thinking cannot simply be avoided, nor should it. Whether it is acknowledged or not, thinking about education issues is always ideologically laden. To claim to be free of ideology is simply not to be aware of its influence. There are dangers in this. As noted earlier, it can lead to an unconscious acceptance of the discursive repertoires associated with one ideological perspective or another. The language of parents as consumers, an undifferentiated group with viewpoints and motivations in common, is one example. The 'core' and 'foundation' subjects of the national curriculum (which exclude other issues which are by definition peripheral or superficial) is a second.

Governments need to be aware, then, that ideology is important in setting the agenda and structuring discourse. Ideology can lead to an emphasis on equality of opportunity and structure the way that phrase is interpreted. Alternatively, it can make such issues invisible. Ideology can lead policy-makers to target particular groups for attention – females, parents, members of minority ethnic groups or teachers – and shape the way they are perceived. Ideology can shape the discursive repertoires that are used, and hence the ways in which education is thought about by the population at large.

New Labour's thinking about education, therefore, is inevitably ideological despite the occasional claims to the contrary. Both the drawbacks and the benefits of ideological thinking need to be taken into account: the limitations, as well as the possibilities for change, need to be appreciated.

Conclusion

This chapter suggests that although Labour has learned a lot about education policy, it continues to have unrealistic expectations of what education can do and has a similarly unrealistic expectation of how far deep-rooted social inequalities can be successfully ameliorated through the educative process. Likewise, the notion that policy-making and legislation are equivalent to achieving the intended outcomes still persists.

However, what Labour has done, in sharp distinction from previous Conservative administrations, is to work to build consensus on its approach to education. In 1990 Ball wrote of the previous Labour administrations: 'There was no attempt by the Labour Party to fashion a broad based national political discourse into which comprehensive education would naturally fit' (Ball 1990a, p. 30). It appears that this is changing as New Labour attempts to establish a vision to which most of the population can subscribe.

Evaluation of the actual policies themselves can be addressed at the technical or the normative levels. At the technical level are questions such as: How practicable were/are these policies? What level of support did or will they elicit from stakeholders? Did or will they achieve their goals? How much waste of resources was or will be involved? How far did they or will they learn from past experience? How relevant were/are they to the needs of those involved? Some of these questions have been addressed in this chapter.

Moving beyond this to the more fundamental normative issues involves the mobilization of political and educational values. Here the issues revolve around not whether the policies will work well, but whether they are the right ones. Questions here include: What has been identified as the 'problem' that needs to be addressed here and what other interpretations are there? Who gains and who loses from this policy? What are the likely consequences, intended and unintended, of this policy for the education system and more broadly? These are left for the reader to judge.

Key points

- While there are marked differences in political ideology and policy-making approaches of New Labour and the New Right, the differences in educational ideology are less distinctive.
- Similarly, while there are many ways in which the educational policies after 1997 were new, there was also continuity in a number of aspects.
- Policy-makers of whichever political complexion tend to make common errors with regard to education policy and appear to be resistant to learning from past mistakes; aspects of policy implementation provide fertile ground in this regard.
- It seems more likely under a New Labour administration than under a New Right one that Britain will begin to adopt some of the characteristics of a 'learning society' which many commentators consider necessary and desirable in the contemporary world.

Guide to further reading

Coffield, F. and Williamson, B. (eds) (1997) *Repositioning Higher Education*, Buckingham: Open University Press/SRHE. This book proposes a new model for higher education based on a critique of current orthodoxies.

Lawton, D. (1992) *Education and Politics in the 1990s: Conflict or Consensus?*, London: Falmer Press. This book looks into the future and includes an interesting discussion on a General Teaching Council, as well as looking at post-compulsory education.

Schuller, T. (ed.) (1995) *The Changing University*, Buckingham: Open University Press/SRHE. This text also looks to the future, including teaching and leadership. Further and higher education are both covered.

For an insight see:

Excellence in Schools White Paper.

This is available at the DfES website (see p. 46). This document clearly sets out the vision for compulsory education which the Labour government had when it entered office and its intentions for turning these into policy. With the benefit of hindsight you will be able to assess the following:

- whether the political tensions inherent in the policy-making process referred to in Chapter 3 resulted in a legislative outcome very different from the vision and policies contained in *Excellence in Schools*
- how far the post-implementation outcomes of that legislation on the ground differed from the intentions expressed in *Excellence in Schools*. That is, was there an 'implementation gap' and if so, what was its size and nature?

Useful websites

http://www.geneseo.edu/~bicket/panop/home.htm

A site called 'k.i.s.s. of the panopticon' (k.i.s.s. stands for 'keep it simple, stupid'. The site itself explains what 'panopticon' means). This is a user-friendly site which explains many of the concepts involved in postmodernism.

www.ncsl.org.uk
The National College for School Leadership

http://ngfl.gov.uk
The National Grid for Learning

Chapter 6
Educational research and education policy

OUTLINE
This chapter sets out two models of the relationship between educational research and education policy: the engineering model and the enlightenment model. It gives examples of both of these, illustrating the diversity of approach within each broad category. Each model is then subjected to critical examination. Finally the key points of the chapter are summarized.

Modelling the relationship between educational research and education policy

In her 1986 book *Research and Policy* Janet Finch makes a distinction between quantitative and qualitative approaches to research. She compares and contrasts the different relationships these have to education policy. This is a useful distinction, but it concentrates on only one aspect of research: the methods of data collection and analysis used. Also it sets up a rather black-and-white set of opposites which, while useful as a way of conceptualizing the relationship between policy and research, does tend to oversimplify the situation.

Developing the idea a little further, we can distinguish between the (social) 'engineering' and the 'enlightenment' models of the relationship between education policy and educational research. Again, this simple binary model masks a number of different perspectives within each category and excludes possible additional categories. However the engineering/enlightenment division at least has the benefit of conceptual clarity, as Table 6.1 illustrates.

Table 6.1 The engineering and enlightenment models of research

	Engineering Model	Enlightenment Model
Type of data collected and analysis method	Bias towards quantitative	Bias towards qualitative
Ontological position (i.e. view of the nature of 'reality')	Foundationalist: considers there to be an objective reality which can be apprehended by research. Research results have a foundation in reality.	Relativist: considers social reality to be socially constructed (to a greater or lesser extent). Research results are true for particular social groups only. They are themselves constructed in nature: stories.
Epistemological position (i.e. view of the status of 'knowledge' created by research)	Absolute/positivist: 'true' knowledge which correctly describes reality can be achieved given sufficient effort and rigour and effort in research.	Relative/interpretative: 'knowledge' is conditional upon its social context. Absolute truths, at least in the social world, are not achievable. Insight and informed judgement are among the important goals of research.
Relationship to policy	Informing policy-makers about the 'facts'. Proposing solutions to 'problems'.	Giving policy-makers enlightenment or challenging the accepted definitions of 'educational problems' and reframing what is problematic in education.

The engineering model

The engineering model adopts a 'scientific' standpoint and a belief that proper, rigorous educational research can give policy-makers hard data and results on which to base their policy decisions. It also implies that it is possible to formulate a rational, top-down, prescription for action on the basis of these decisions. It is linked, in other words, to the managerial approach to policy implementation discussed in Chapter 4. In this view the role of educational research is to explain how the educational world works and to suggest action. Early work in this category is sometimes described as being in the 'political arithmetic' tradition of 'objective' methods of data collection and analysis used to inform political choices. Early social reformers in this tradition included Booth and Rowntree, who studied the nature and extent of poverty, as well as (later) Glass and Halsey, who studied social mobility and education.

One example of how research and policy-making can be linked in this way is in the work of the Robbins Committee on higher education (1963). The Committee commissioned a large programme of research, comprising six major surveys of students, lecturers and young people, as well as several smaller studies. A famous statistician acted as adviser to the Committee and all the research they relied on was quantitative in character. Much use was made of these data in justifying the recommendations of the Committee, which called for an accelerated expansion in higher education provision.

Another example of this approach is the 'Three Wise Men' report (Alexander et al. 1992). This arose out of the appointment by Kenneth Clarke (then the Conservative Education Secretary) of three leading academics whose task was to review the current state of primary education and to make recommendations. The authors were given only a few months to do their work and, partly for this reason, did not conduct any original research, confining themselves instead to a review of the available literature. Their report was published in January 1992 and was sent to local education authorities, teacher training institutions and elsewhere. The 'Three Wise Men's' conclusions were that, although there was much to commend in primary schools, there was too much 'patchiness' in standards between and within schools, and that teachers needed to be more systematic in their planning and to create a better balance between whole-class and individualized teaching strategies. A key paragraph contained the following words:

> Teachers will need to abandon the [progressivist] dogma of recent decades. They will need to focus firmly on the outcomes

of their teaching . . . They will need to direct close attention to
the balance of whole class, group and individual teaching
strategies . . . [and of] . . . subject and topic teaching.
(Alexander et al. 1992, p. 49)

The report was sent out with a press release from the DES
entitled *'Three Wise Men' Report Calls for Big Changes in Primary
Education.* This emphasized the Report's criticisms of 'highly
questionable dogmas' and stressed that topic work had led to
'fragmentary and superficial teaching and learning', that there was
not enough whole-class teaching being done, and that grouping by
subject ability was a desirable strategy.

The quotation from Kenneth Clarke in the press release emphasized the need for 'fundamental changes' in primary education
and that although all of the proposals were 'being practiced [*sic*]
somewhere in the country', not enough schools were following what
was now known to be best practice. The 'wise men' themselves
and Kenneth Clarke assumed that the report presented a definitive
account of 'the facts' about primary school practice and could be
used as a guide for all teachers throughout the country.

The need for a greater linkage of research and policy

From the engineering perspective it is a sad fact that there has only
been at best a loose linkage between educational research and
education policy. There are five main reasons for this.

Research fads

First, the topics focused on by the research community have not
always been much use to policy-makers. The topics researchers
pursue tend to be driven not only by the funding available but
by academic and publishing trends. At the moment, for example,
ethnic disadvantage in education is hot, social class inequality is
not. Globalization, postmodernism and personal identity are in,
classroom interaction studies are out.

Jargon

Second, researchers frequently do not speak a language that is accessible to policy-makers and others. Few researchers seem to take account of effective dissemination of research results to policy-makers. The same is true of communication with practitioners: a study by Dai Hounsell et al. (1980) showed that most teachers (82 per cent) felt that there was a gulf between teachers and researchers, with 44 per cent of teachers poorly informed about educational research and development. Most (86 per cent) felt that research reports are tedious to read, with too much jargon (70 per cent) and not often communicated to schools (81 per cent.) Around 40 per cent felt that researchers were not really interested in or informed about topics that were relevant to teachers. According to Hargreaves (1996) and Tooley and Darby (1998) the situation had not improved nearly twenty years later.

Politicians' suspicions about researchers

Third, politicians often distrust educational researchers, seeing them as simply another self-interested lobby. Kenneth Clarke is reported to have said that researchers rarely reach any other conclusion than that more research is needed.

Poor-quality research

Fourth, from an engineering model point of view, there is the current inadequacy of the social sciences to gather data and test theory in the kinds of reliable and verifiable ways that the natural sciences do these things.

The political nature of policy-making

Perhaps more important, however, is the fact that political ideologies and the micro-politics of policy-making are often more important in policy formulation than a rational consideration of the results of evaluative and other forms of research. This certainly appears to have been the case with the academic evaluation of the pilots of records of achievement in schools, as well as evaluations of educational vouchers, even when these were conducted in-house (Department of Employment 1992; James 1993).

An impossible dream?

Critics of the engineering model would claim that even if all five of the points above were somehow nullified, the engineering model could never work. There are three main reasons for this.

It is not possible to find 'the truth'

The engineering model assumes that it is possible for educational research to establish 'the truth' and the 'correct' way of doing things in schools, colleges and universities. There are a number of problems with these assumptions. First, any research study will inevitably be selective, focusing on some issues and ignoring others. The partial nature of research means that conclusions will also be partial: a particular 'take' on reality, rather than a full depiction of it. Critics of the 'Three Wise Men' Report argue that the 'wise men's' selection and interpretation of the evidence was heavily conditioned by the political climate in which they were operating. This had led to the selection of these three researchers rather than others, and these particular people were influenced in their selection and interpretation of the data they examined by their own pre-existing viewpoints. Second, social contexts which, on the face of it, appear very similar are in fact very different from each other. Research conclusions which may apply in one, for example in a primary school, may be very wide of the mark in another, even another primary school. As was noted in Chapter 5, educational settings in particular differ in very important ways, so that any attempt to establish a widely generalizable 'truth' is flawed.

Educational research and 'interested parties'

A linked issue which affects educational research in particular is that it, like education policy, is highly contested terrain. As with education policy, individuals, groups and organizations with different agendas are often keen to be involved in shaping and interpreting research issues, approaches and outcomes.

Although we do not know for sure the grounds upon which the 'Three Wise Men' were selected by the Conservative government, it is clear that they were well known as critics of 'progressivism'. Robin Alexander, for example, had conducted earlier research in Leeds primary schools which was heavily critical of 'progressive' methods there; this received national publicity on television as well as being published as a report and book (Alexander 1992a). Another of the three, Chris Woodhead, later to become the head of the HMI service and at the time Chief Executive of the National Curriculum Council, was an outspoken critic of the teaching profession, and very unpopular among teachers for being the mouthpiece of the government's attack upon them. It is possible to surmise, then, that the government knew what it wanted the report to say and chose the authors on that basis.

There is also an increasing tendency for the terms of funded contract research to be very tightly drawn by the commissioning agency. The methodology and timetabling of the research may be so closely set by the contractor that some researchers feel they are simply 'delivering' goods in an unreflective (and uncritical) way as if the sponsor was 'contracting for ten tons of aggregate . . . or buying a fridge' (Pettigrew 1994, p. 44). Most worrying, however, are attempts by sponsors to delay, suppress or change results. 'About three years ago you started to get comments back [on draft research reports] from "there should be a full stop there" to "take that out, it is contrary to government policy"' (quoted in Pettigrew 1994, p. 45).

Although researchers too are motivated by interests and sometimes hidden agendas, there is likely to be more diversity in values and attitudes among educational researchers than in sponsoring agencies. If there is creeping manipulation of educational research by interested parties, then the engineering model's ideal of policy-makers using 'objective' results from disinterested research fades away. This problem is compounded by the fact that the dissemination of research results through the mass media is not impartial. The gloss placed upon the 'Three Wise Men' Report by the DES press release which accompanied it was picked up by the mass media which, on the whole, accepted the DES interpretation of the Report as rejecting all aspects of progressivism out of hand. Alexander was so concerned about the way the Report was publicly interpreted that he went so far as to write a rebuttal of this interpretation (Alexander 1992b). Like education policy, educational research reports are not received in a vacuum but in a context highly charged with competing interests and value systems.

Putting conclusions into practice

The engineering model assumes that research reports can be translated unproblematically into action. But, however they are presented to their eventual audiences, the latter will filter those findings through their own preconceptions, values and attitudes. In this sense, too, there is a parallel between policy research and policy implementation. In both cases 'text' is 'read' in an active way by highly differentiated audiences. Teachers, for example, will not simply react to research reports in an automatic way, but will selectively interpret them and decide to act, not to act or to change their practice in unpredictable ways.

There is a further problem within the simplistic linkage between research and policy set up by the engineering model. It contains the assumption that in both teaching and educational management it is possible to lift simple solutions from a well-researched 'toolbox' of techniques and answers – the notion of 'evidence-based practice'. This is fundamentally misguided. Good classroom teaching involves a sense of appropriate and inappropriate teacher behaviour which is finely attuned to subtleties of context, group dynamics and pupil personality. Split-second decisions are made, based on tacit knowledge in a very skilled way. In short, teachers need to be reflective practitioners whose behaviour, while informed by research, is also largely shaped by professional experience and local knowledge. No matter how good the research or reliable the findings, educational contexts are always going to differ from each other in important ways. The good teacher or educational manager will always need to develop a keen sense of how to deal with this unpredictability.

The enlightenment model

The aim of this approach is to illuminate educational issues, giving policy-makers a good grounding in the context within which they seek to make policy, including well-formulated theories and concepts which can make it more explicable to them. There is no attempt to deliver 'the truth', because that is seen as a fundamentally problematic concept. However, it is important that policy-makers should be aware of the different versions of the truth that are relevant in the policy field they are considering, because these have important implications for policy outcomes. In this sense the enlightenment model is closely allied to the phenomenological perspective on the implementation of change (see Chapter 4).

As with the engineering approach, a variety of types of research fit under this heading, including ethnographic and evaluative work. Parlett and Hamilton, for example, wrote a famous paper in 1972 entitled 'Evaluation as illumination' which set out a new approach to evaluative research, and triggered a shift away from the engineering model. Instead Parlett and Hamilton advocated adopting an 'anthropological' research approach, in which the programme being evaluated, including its rationale, operation, achievements and difficulties, is studied intensively. A fuller understanding is achieved by studying the subject intensively and in context.

Action research involves the attempt to improve professional practice through research. Some forms of this belong in the enlightenment category. The *practical approach* (Kemmis 1993) seeks to enlighten teachers and others (parents, students), by giving them responsibility for the policy outcomes which follow research, the research being conducted jointly between them and academics. *Emancipatory action research* seeks to empower teachers and others, by giving them full responsibility for research and any changes in practice which follow it. This is perhaps the most elaborated example of the relationship between research and policy in education within the enlightenment tradition.

From the point of view of *critical social research* (Troyna 1994), the task should be critical theorizing rather than just problem-solving. The problem-solving approach takes the world as given, including the current power relationships and structured disadvantage. From a critical social research point of view, action research which accepts the status quo is effectively supporting it because it is attempting to make it work more smoothly. Critical social research rejects this, and aims to raise awareness of the inequalities and injustices inherent in current social arrangements in the hope of ultimately changing them.

Critical social theorists, for example, argue that the school improvement and school effectiveness strands of educational research have two important limitations.

- They assume that, given the right technical fixes within any school (changes in management styles, and in teaching and assessment methods), then all children can succeed regardless of their background. Such an approach makes invisible the linkages between schooling and issues of social class, disability, gender and ethnicity, and generally the structured nature of advantage and disadvantage in the British education system (Ball 1990a; Angus 1993; Whitty 1997).
- These research approaches have been captured by New Right and New Labour discourse in that they implicitly accept the model of schools as autonomous units which can, through self-help, improve themselves in a competitive environment. In reality, the 'competition' between schools takes place on a playing field which is far from level, with some schools disadvantaged in terms of funding, the cultural capital possessed by pupils in their catchment area, and in many other ways.

By contrast, critical social research aims:

- to situate issues in their social context
- to promote radical change through critically addressing, rather than accepting, current policies and practices
- to take account of the political, ideological and discursive struggles which surround education policy-making.

From this point of view, key issues for educational research in the policy field in the twenty-first century include:

- the investigation of how educational reforms impact on class, gender, 'race' and disability, both in the education professions and among students

- the investigation of the nature and impact of equal opportunities policies in educational institutions and more broadly
- the evaluation of the impact of changes in teacher training and professional development for teachers and managers (e.g. on women)
- the investigation into the consequences, intended and un-intended, of curriculum and other 'reforms', particularly on the already disadvantaged
- working for change and improvement by, for example, challenging the discursive practices which limit our ability to visualize and express alternatives: Ball's (1995) 'semiotic guerrilla warfare'.

Case study: scheming for youth

David Lee and a team of researchers conducted a research project lasting six years into the government-funded youth training scheme (YTS) in a town in the south-east of England which they called 'Southwich'. YTS was designed to help get school leavers into work by giving them the skills needed in employment, by providing formal education in college linked to government-funded placement with an employer. The research funded by the Leverhulme Trust aimed to evaluate the effectiveness of this scheme. The research methods used included collecting background statistical data, administering two consecutive written questionnaires to school leavers, and conducting almost two hundred interviews with young people on youth training schemes.

While the authors agree that 'British schooling has for too long been impoverished by rigid and elitist ideas of academic worth', their study concludes that youth training in the form it took at that time did not solve the problem. They found that trainees complained that they were being prepared for 'Noddy jobs'. The trainees' comments illustrate this: ' "All I learned was how to make the tea. . . . I used to pick up loads of potatoes and coal and load the lorry. I got all sweaty and dirty. The reason they wanted me was as a sort of dogsbody" ' (Lee et al. 1990, p. 166). Only one trainee, in a hospital, felt that she was receiving proper training, but she faced the hostility of NHS auxiliaries who felt that she represented 'cheap labour' filling the place of one of their number.

The researchers also found that the youth training experience was not itself marketable to employers. In some cases it even had a stigma attached to it, so that the trainee's chance of getting a job was worse after than before the 'training'. Although a relatively high proportion of the trainees whom they studied did get jobs after the scheme, they were often in low-status or unskilled occupations. The main contribution to any job-hunting success the trainees had appeared to come from the fact that employers were using the scheme as a probationary period for potential new staff.

More fundamentally, however, the researchers concluded that:

> the emphasis of the scheme upon so-called 'free-market forces' severely limits its effectiveness as a means of training young workers and providing them with opportunities to improve their personal circumstances through paid work.
>
> (Lee et al. 1990, p. ix)

The neo-liberal underpinnings of the scheme were its fundamental flaw. In these authors' view market forces cannot compensate for fundamental social inequalities, they only magnify their effects.

> The more unregulated are market forces, the more difficult it becomes to provide the kind of skill training that will upgrade the long-term capabilities and living standards of the workforce. Nor will market forces do much to eradicate the costly social insecurities in young workers' home lives which decrease their ability and willingness to learn be taught.
>
> (Lee et al. 1990, p. 192)

Because the Manpower Services Commission (MSC), which oversaw the scheme, lacked much power, thanks to this free market philosophy, it could not, despite its good intentions, intervene to limit employers' behaviour which reinforced the gendered nature of occupational recruitment, thus again reinforcing existing social inequalities.

> It is an irony imposed by market forces, that a scheme with the formal goal of equal opportunities became a finely-graded

sieve for matching young people to placements with very unequal job prospects and levels of skills training.

(Lee et al. 1990, p. 63)

Moreover it is wrong, the authors argue, to equate the interests and behaviour of employers with the public good.

It is useless in a system whose whole rationale is based on short-term competitive individualism to expect hard-pressed employers to behave altruistically with an eye to the long-term public interest . . . Individual employers will only invest in workers they intend to use for their own production needs.

(Lee et al. 1990, pp. 192–3)

Lee et al.'s report concludes by arguing that the government should 'seek ways of protecting training from market forces by all means in their power' (p. 193). Training standards within individual firms need to be regulated by public bodies with teeth, they argue, and unions and young people need to be represented on those bodies. Also important is raising the general educational standard of young people and encouraging more young people to continue longer in post-compulsory education. To encourage this vocational education should offer a ladder of progression, not just short-term schemes. Finally employers, managers and training supervisors need to be educated about the value of scholarship and science because they place too much emphasis on the 'practical', in the view of these authors. The authors conclude with the following paragraph.

The real 'immorality' of YTS lies with a [Conservative] government so blinded by its own rhetoric of the 'enterprise culture' that it is prepared to conceal the scheme's failure and to exclude young people from their basic rights if they refuse to join. Until they provide adequate funds and regulation, government ministers should stop making bogus claims that all YTS provides quality training.

(Lee et al. 1990, p. 195)

Some problems

The link between research and policy

The nature of the link between research and policy is less clear in enlightenment research than in the engineering model. Ethnographic work only rarely ends with a section on the policy implications of the research. Lee et al.'s study is an exception. It combines a critique of neo-liberalism with an outline of an alternative. However, the proposals are couched in the most general terms.

Generalizability

Enlightenment research has been accused of producing findings which are non-cumulative: a series of interesting but essentially non-comparable case studies. Some enlightenment theorists argue that this is inevitable.

> The interpretivist rejects generalisation as a goal and never aims to draw randomly selected samples of human experience. For the interpretivist every instance of social interaction, if thickly described (Geertz 1973), represents a slice from the life world that is the proper subject matter for interpretive inquiry . . . Every topic . . . must be seen as carrying its own logic, sense of order, structure and meaning.
>
> (Denzin 1983, pp. 133–4)

Understandably, such a position is unlikely to give policy-makers confidence in the research findings, since it is unclear whether or not they apply in most, some or even any of the cases to which the proposed policy might apply.

Qualitative research is often ignored by policy-makers

Enlightenment research appears to be largely ignored by government, while the social engineering approach, with its quantitative methods, has had considerable impact on education policy. There are a number of possible explanations for this.

- Statistical data are more useful to government; they enable the government to classify the population and institutions hierarchically and 'manage' them, distinguishing, for example, the deserving from the undeserving. The use of school league tables is one example of this. According to many Marxist, feminist and other conflict perspectives this is a major function of government policy-making.

- Empiricism and positivism have traditionally higher status in the UK than qualitative approaches, at least among the population at large. Policy-makers and others are suspicious of research not based on large samples and claiming to be generalizable. Moreover, policy-makers tend to adopt an unproblematic attitude towards 'facts' and feel that they are more easily able to evaluate the quality of research in the positivist tradition.

- Educational research in general and qualitative research in particular is seen as partisan, in particular as biased towards the left, by policy-makers. There are suspicions about bias in the conduct of research and the presentation of findings. Poor sampling, unsubstantiated arguments and the selective use of evidence and secondary sources renders much of this research virtually valueless, according to one OFSTED-published report (Tooley and Darby 1998). Despite robust refutations of such views (Hammersley 2000), these suspicions tend to linger.

However, Angela McRobbie (1994) notes that the influence of research studies on policy can be more subtle than a simple call for or reference to research results during the policy-making process. She argues that the expansion of higher education, and the fact that upper-level policy-makers are nowadays very likely to have a degree, often in the social sciences, means that a general understanding of theories and concepts and evidence accumulated in social science research has already permeated the culture to such an extent that it influences policy in an 'invisible' way. Perhaps it is in this way that qualitative research is most likely to have an effect on policy-making.

Ethical issues

Research in the enlightenment tradition tends to raise ethical issues more frequently than engineering research does. Because it is closer to the subjects of the research, and more revealing about them, a tension is created between the need to disclose in order to achieve greater illumination and the need to conceal in order to protect the subjects of research. In such instances the researcher is in a double bind: anonymizing the context and withholding or changing information about it undermines external observers' ability to check findings and raises doubts about the validity and reliability of the research; but complete openness puts respondents in jeopardy.

Key points

- The link between research and policy can usually be viewed from within one of two paradigms: the engineering model or the enlightenment model.
- The engineering model is aligned to the top-down, managerial model of policy implementation, while the enlightenment model is closer to the phenomenological perspective on change (see Chapter 4) because of the insights it gives into the cultures of actors on the ground.
- Each paradigm has a very different conception of appropriate aims, methodologies, methods and aspirations in education policy research and of the nature of the link between research and policy.
- Each has its own unique set of strengths and weaknesses. To date, policy-makers have tended to give more credence to research founded upon engineering approaches, despite their numerous weaknesses.
- However, policy-making and the reception of research findings are both complicated processes. The rational appraisal of research findings and their subsequent seamless integration into the policy-making process rarely happens. Policy-making is more usually driven by political negotiation and compromise than by the cool appraisal of available evidence. Similarly, research

results are received, interpreted and filtered by segmented audiences whose perception of them is largely conditioned by their pre-existing ideological and cultural characteristics.

Guide to further reading

For good edited volumes covering a number of key issues see:

Burgess, R. (ed.) (1993) *Educational Research and Evaluation for Policy and Practice?*, London: Falmer Press.

Halpin, D. and Troyna, B. (eds) (1994) *Researching Education Policy: Ethical and Methodological Issues*, London: Falmer Press.

Hammersley, M. (ed.) (1993) *Educational Research: Current Issues*, Buckingham: Open University Press and Paul Chapman Publishing.

For important journal papers see:

Troyna, B. (1994) 'Critical Social Research and Education Policy', *British Journal of Educational Studies*, 42, 1, pp. 70–84. This whole issue of *British Journal of Educational Studies* carries a number of important papers, including Stephen Ball's guest editorial: 'At the Crossroads: Education Policy Studies', as well as Fitz et al.'s 'Implementation Research and Education Policy: Practice and Prospects'.

For an insight see:

James, M. 'Evaluation for Policy: Rationality and Political Reality: the Paradigm Case of PRAISE?', in R. Burgess (ed.) (1993) *Educational Research and Evaluation for Policy and Practice*, London: Falmer Press, pp. 119–38. This provides a brief readable account of commissioned research into government policy on records of achievement (RoAs). In 1985 what became the Pilot Records of Achievement in Schools Evaluation (PRAISE) team was commissioned by the Department for Education and Science to evaluate the pilot schemes of recording achievement that had been set up. RoAs involved pupils compiling, with their teachers, statements of what they had experienced and achieved in school and outside it, as well as identifying areas for their own personal development and planning for the future. The £10 million PRAISE project was designed to evaluate how far the aims of recording achievement (which included improving the recognition of achievement, increasing pupils' motivation and personal development, improving curriculum and organization and providing a document of record) were being fulfilled. The article gives an account of the political tensions surrounding RoAs which illustrate well some of the points made in Chapter 3 about 'encoding policy'. It also shows how these spilled over into the PRAISE project and evaluates how far the data and conclusions which derived from the PRAISE were important in the development of RoA policy. The RoA example is generally an interesting case study of the link between policy and research, partly because so much has been written about it, partly because it arouses strength of feeling among critics and supporters, and partly because of the fact that there has been a considerable amount of research on the issue, both commissioned and independent. Some of this is discussed in Trowler and Hinett (1994), which also contains an extensive bibliography on the issue. This article is available in full on the Web at: http://www.lle.mdx.ac.uk/hec/journal/1-1/2-4.htm.

Useful website

http://www.lancs.ac.uk/staff/trowler/ressite/
designed for those involved or simply interested in educational research.

Glossary

Action research: Small-scale involvement in the world, using research methods to study the effects of actions and making changes based on the results. In most cases it is practitioner research, that is, it is done by people investigating their own professional practices, and the methods used are often qualitative in character. Elliott (1991) sums up a key feature of action research when he says that 'action research is about improving practice rather than producing knowledge'.

Banding: Division of the year group into two, three or four bands, differentiated by ability on criteria similar to those used for streaming; each band contains a number of classes, not necessarily of equal ability or size (Harlen and Malcolm 1997).

Black Papers: Written by members of the right who mounted a sustained critique of the British education system between 1969 and 1977. There were three main themes:

- Academic standards, particularly numeracy and literacy, are in decline.
- Politically motivated teachers represent a danger both in the classroom and outside it, because they espouse progressive teaching and assessment methods, as well as feminist and socialist ideology, and are fundamentally opposed to industrialism and vocationalism in education.
- Indiscipline is increasing in schools and threatens to disrupt the fabric of society.

Butskellism: Combination of the names of 'Rab' Butler and Hugh Gaitskell, senior Conservative and Labour figures respectively. The word signifies the postwar settlement between the two parties on issues such as nationalization, education and social policy during the period roughly between 1944 and 1976.

Conflict perspectives: Views which see society as divided into two or more groups whose interests are intrinsically opposed. The category covers a variety of Marxist perspectives, as well as a range of feminisms. Marxism sees society as inevitably divided into competitive classes, one of which owns the means of production (land, factories, etc.), and the other which does not. Human history is largely driven by the clash between the opposing classes. Education helps maintain the dominance of certain powerful groups in society. Feminist perspectives have been classified into liberal, radical, socialist and black feminism, though such a classification system has been criticized on a number of grounds (van Zoonen 1994). Each has in common the view that women have been systematically disadvantaged by a patriarchal society. Feminists point to the fact that patriarchy is reproduced in the education system in a number of ways. Conflict perspectives call for a clear differentiation between policy rhetoric and the reality of policy outcomes: the actual effects of policy on disadvantaged groups or those discriminated against, such as minority ethnic groups, women and those from socio-economically deprived backgrounds. Understanding the ideological provenance of policy and the operation of hegemony, i.e. dominant ways of seeing the world and talking about it, is also important from these perspectives. Education policy is largely seen as encapsulating the interests and world view of privileged groups, whether consciously or not, and it is necessary for those committed to change to work against this.

Corporate culturalism: Approaches to the management of change which stress the manipulation of organizational culture by senior management for the achievement of corporate goals.

Council for National Academic Awards (CNAA):   This body regulated degrees awarded by the polytechnics. It was abolished in 1992 with the abolition of the binary divide.

Cultural capital: Bourdieu argues that there are three forms of cultural capital: the embodied state, the objectified state and the institutionalized state (Bourdieu 1997, p. 47). The 'embodied state' of cultural capital refers to 'long-lasting dispositions of mind and body'. Examples might include any of the cultural resources that are valuable in achieving educational success, such as self-confidence, the ability to defer certain sorts of gratification, modes of speech and thought, and so on. 'Objectified cultural capital' is that which is translated into transmissible material objects. The 'institutionalized state' of cultural capital is one form of this: 'the objectification of cultural capital in the form of academic qualifications' (Bourdieu 1997, p. 50). Each of these can be transformed into the others in the same way that other forms of capital (economic, social) can be transformed ('transubstantiated') into cultural capital and vice versa. When pupils enter school or students enter university with a considerable amount of accumulated cultural capital, then the institution's task is easier and the chances of 'success' higher.

DES/DfE/DfEE/DfES: The name of the government department responsible for education has changed over the years from the Department of Education and Science (DES), to the Department for Education (DfE), to the Department for Education and Employment (DfEE) and Department for Education and Skills (DfES) most recently.

Dirigisme: State control of economic and social matters.

Fordism: An approach to the management of production, originally of cars, which involves the following characteristics:

- de-skilling
- the equalization of wage rates at a relatively high level
- intensification of work and the predetermination of work output
- the automatic movement of work between workers
- the employment of those capable of doing the job, but no more
- the extension of control outside the factory (or other site of 'production')
- mass production of a standard product for a very large market (Watkins 1994).

Some writers argue that aspects of the Fordist approach are now being applied in education. Others argue that we are now seeing a 'neo-Fordist' or 'post-Fordist' phase in the organization of education. The term 'neo-Fordism' suggests that delivery is organized along managerialist lines (see **Managerialism** below) and it shares with Fordism an emphasis on quick, cheap delivery of a product which meets market demand. 'Post-Fordism' implies that the organization of production is conducted in an extremely flexible way to meet the twin challenge of limited resources and a fast-changing market. Staff are employed on short-term and part-time contracts in the main or as 'consultants'. Production rates and the products themselves are changed with great rapidity.

Functionalism: The dominant sociological approach both in the UK and the USA in the 1950s and 1960s. Functionalism is a perspective which sees social organization as possessing many similarities to the physical make-up of an animal's body. Both the body and society consist of distinguishable parts (legs, eyes, etc., for the one, the church, family, etc., for the other). In both animals and society the parts all play some clear role, i.e. they fulfil a function (movement, sight, etc., social integration, human reproduction, etc.). In both, too, the different parts act together to form a system which (usually) operates smoothly to fulfil the goals of the whole. Functionalism, as applied to the study of education, takes the view that the contents of the school curriculum should reflect and propagate the common culture. The role of the teacher is to transmit this common culture; the teacher acts as a jug from which the dominant norms and values of society are poured into the empty vessels in the classroom.

Policy-makers often operate on an implicit functionalist model when making policy: education is seen as being able to perform important functions in society as a whole, particularly in fostering greater integration and improved economic efficiency, while reducing crime and deviance. This rather simple set of assumptions leads them into common errors, as the discussion in Chapter 5 indicated. At the level of the management of change in the individual school or college, functionalist thinking has likewise led to simplistic thinking about organizational culture which sees it as enacted by individuals in a puppet-like way, and as being relatively easily manipulable by managers in order to effect desired changes. A strong, unitary culture is seen as highly functional for educational institutions, and managers strive to achieve this in order to bring about change.

Grant-maintained (GM) school: School which has opted out of local authority control by balloting parents and which receives funding directly from a government agency. It has more autonomy than a maintained school.

Implementation gap: The differences between the intended outcomes of policy as originally envisaged by policy-makers, and those which were actually realized after the policy had been implemented.

Implementation staircase: The various levels or sites, national, regional and local, at which education policy is received, interpreted and put into practice, sometimes in ways which are quite different from those originally intended by policy-makers.

Local Education Authority (LEA): The part of local government at the county level or equivalent responsible for aspects of education in its area.

Local management of schools (LMS): A shorthand way of referring to the devolution of powers to schools' governing bodies to look after more of their own affairs. Conversely powers have been lost by LEAs with this development.

Maintained school: School maintained by the state, as opposed to a private school or one maintained by, for example, the church.

Managerialism: 'A set of beliefs and practices, at the core of which burns the seldom tested assumption that better management will prove an effective solvent for a wide range of economic and social ills' (Pollitt 1990). Its practices include the following:

- strict financial management and devolved budgetary controls
- the efficient use of resources and the emphasis on productivity
- the extensive use of quantitative performance indicators
- the development of consumerism and the discipline of the market

- the manifestation of consumer charters as mechanisms for accountability
- the creation of a disciplined, flexible workforce, using flexible or individualized contracts, staff appraisal systems and performance-related pay
- the assertion of managerial control and the managers' right to manage (Randle and Brady 1997).

Manpower Services Commission (MSC):   An arm of the Employment Department when this was separate from the Education Department, it intervened in education policy, sometimes in competition with the DES. It was later renamed a number of times and eventually became TEED: the Training, Enterprise and Education Directorate. It controls the work of local TECs (Training and Enterprise Councils) which are concerned with vocational education and training at the regional level.

Multiple cultural configuration in organisations (MCC):   The 'multiple cultural configuration' (Alvesson 2002) approach to organizations such as schools and universities, which can be contrasted to the functionalist one. While functionalism sees their cultures as homogeneous and coherent, shared by everyone, the MCC approach sees every school, at least large ones, as having numerous subcultures of different levels and kinds. People derive attitudes, values and ways of behaving from their gender, class, ethnicity, from their location in the school (teacher, student, head) and from the wider society. These cultures overlap in the school or university and are influenced by its particular character. 'Cultural traffic' moves around within the organization, the traffic flow being shaped by the issues being addressed at any particular time and the ideologies that are relevant to them. Conflict, sometimes open and sometimes under-the-stage, is the norm. In contrast the functionalist view sees agreement and stability as characterizing a healthy school, university or other organization. From the MCC perspective change is constant as the cultural traffic shifts around new issues and as new influences flow into the organization. From the functionalist viewpoint stability is the norm. The two approaches have very different implications for the understanding of policy implementation.

National Commission on Education: Funded by the Paul Hamlyn Foundation, this group of 'the great and the good' conducted an extensive investigation into education in the UK. It published *Learning to Succeed* (1993), *Learning to Succeed After Sixteen* (1995), *Learning to Succeed: The Way Ahead* (1995) and *Success Against the Odds* (1996). Despite their unofficial status, these publications both reflected and influenced educational thought in the mid-1990s.

National Council for Vocational Qualifications (NCVQ): Quango created in 1986 and charged with establishing a common, coherent framework for vocational qualifications. This has developed into the system of national vocational qualifications (NVQs). NCVQ also created general national vocational qualifications (GNVQs). See also **Qualifications and Curriculum Authority (QCA)**.

OFSTED: the Office for Standards in Education. This organization was set up to improve standards of achievement in state-funded schools in England. It uses regular school inspections and public reporting of its findings to do this. OFSTED's website is at http://www.ofsted.gov.uk.

Phenomenology: Traditionally, sociology pictures individuals as being born into a world over which they have no real control; society is something that does things to people. The phenomenological perspective, founded by Husserl (1931), replaces this essentially passive view of humankind with a view that stresses people's autonomy in creating their social world, viewing reality as at least partly socially constructed. Phenomenologists are interested in people's 'taken for granted' reality: their everyday recurrent practices, the ways in which they define the situation they are in and the way they understand their world in general. However, this is a sociological perspective rather than an individual psychological one because social processes are important in shaping individual's understandings. Schutz, Husserl's pupil, for example, stresses that subjective meanings and motives are shared and understood by everyone in a given society: 'typifications' of situations and behaviour, shared by the actors involved, are very important mechanisms for sustaining coherence in social interaction. Phenomenology is important in understanding policy-making and policy interpretation and the relationship between them; it shows us that neither policy-makers nor policy implementers should be viewed as homogenous groups, but in a more subtle way, as people who will perceive the meanings of policy statements differently and will have different definitions of the situation in which policy is being made and implemented.

Policy as discourse: Refers to the idea that the ways in which policy is expressed and the areas it focuses on (and ignores) structure the ways in which policy is (and is not) thought about.

Policy as text: It is necessary to distinguish between formal statements of policy found in documents and seeing policy as text. When seen as 'text', policies are viewed as statements which can be understood and interpreted ('read') in different ways depending upon the audience and the context. This idea is elaborated more fully in Chapter 4.

Policy culture: 'The structures and policy goals, and dominant discourses and practices within public bureaucracies which frame the possibilities for policy' (Lingard and Garrick 1997, p. 2).

Policy refraction: The distortion of policy which takes place as a result of the interaction of competing interests and sets of values. Policy becomes disjointed and less coherent as it goes through the 'encoding' and 'decoding' processes: it is refracted (Taylor et al. 1997, p. 119).

Policy trajectory (study): Policy trajectory refers to the different phases of policy-making and implementation, from the genesis of an idea underlying a policy development to its being put into practice in educational institutions (for example). A policy trajectory study is one which conducts research into each aspect of a policy's trajectory. Ball makes the point that the analytical consequences of a dual understanding of policy, as both text and as discourse, is to conduct what he calls policy trajectory studies. By this he means studies which trace the progress of policy from its formulation stage (where struggles, interpretations and compromises are mapped) through to the recipients of policy at the ground level (where interpretations and implementation strategies are similarly mapped). The policy trajectory research strategy holds out the prospect of a much fuller, more rounded, understanding of the processes and outcomes of education policy-making and implementation, of the constraining effects of the environment, as well as the power of actors.

Postmodernism and personal identity: Postmodernism is a social theory which argues that the social world has reached a condition of postmodernity. Here there is a free flow of information on a global scale and people are no longer rooted to their locale. Many contrasting sources of information are available to individuals and they are able to pick and choose from them. In this way they are empowered to create their own identity, which becomes increasingly fluid, and to construct the social world in which they live by choosing from the myriad styles and possibilities available to them. Consumption, in this very wide sense, is an important feature of postmodernity. Meanwhile, there is a loss of faith in the ability of science, religion or any other 'grand narrative' to achieve any meaningful truth or answers. Individuals are cast on to their own resources; what is right for them and the communities they choose to inhabit is right, full stop. There are, however, constraints on individuals' power. An important one of these is the discursive repertoires available to them. From a postmodernist point of view the language we use, the discourse, both represents reality and creates it; it structures the way we think, and can think, about the world. This has an important significance in thinking about education policy; the discursive devices used in framing policy may make thinking about alternatives difficult or impossible. The policy medium thus may be as important as its message, or even be the message. Hargreaves and Reynolds (1989) show how the discourse of the national curriculum has excluded other curricular possibilities from consideration, for example. The postmodernist view of the modern world also has more general consequences for the consideration of education policy. From this perspective our whole approach to education at all levels is based on outmoded 'modernist' thinking and needs to be completely reconsidered.

Qualifications and Curriculum Authority (QCA): Quango created in October 1997 from the merger of NCVQ (National Council for Vocational Qualifications) and SCAA (School Curriculum and Assessment Authority) (see next entry). QCA is the regulatory body responsible for the national curriculum and for all academic and vocational qualifications in England and Wales below the level of first degrees. It has very substantial powers.

School Curriculum and Assessment Authority (SCAA): Quango responsible for the national curriculum and for GCSEs and AS/A levels. See also **Qualifications and Curriculum Authority (QCA).**

School effectiveness and school improvement research: Two linked strands of research which attempt to identify the characteristics of good schools and successful approaches to managing school improvement, usually through quantitative research. They both fall into the 'engineering' category of the link between research and policy. See, for example, Reynolds and Cuttance (1992) and Ainscow et al. (1994).

Setting: The regrouping of pupils according to their ability in the subject concerned. This can be carried out across the whole year group or within a band or population, provided that two or more classes can be timetabled for the same subject at the same time. Setting can therefore be used within any pattern or organization. Schools frequently seek to make teaching groups smaller and more homogeneous by providing extra sets, for example by regrouping the ninety pupils in three classes into four or five sets, although staffing constraints make it unlikely that this can be done in more than a few subjects (Harlen and Malcolm 1997).

Streaming: The method of assigning pupils to classes on some overall assessment of general ability, the most able pupils in one stream, the next most able in the next, and so on. The classes so streamed are used as the teaching units for the majority of subjects (Harlen and Malcolm 1997).

Structuration theory: Structuration theory tries to find a compromise between the theory of society which says that people's behaviour is rigidly controlled by the social groups they live in (the kind of structuralism seen in functionalism, for example), and the idea that they are free to construct their own realities (the action theory on which phenomenology is based). For many theorists these positions are too extreme. Structuration theory as developed by Tony Giddens says that, while structures are important in conditioning the way people think and behave, these structures are not external to thought and behaviour. They can be changed and often are, sometimes as a result of conscious decisions by people and sometimes in an unconscious way. Structures and action are both important, each is implicit in the other. The sophistication of Giddensian structuration theory lies in this insight that structure and action are interdependent and mutually causative, so that good social theory must appreciate both. People behave in consistent ways, patterned and influenced by the structural contexts in which they live, by ideologies, cultures, and so on. At the same time they create their social world and alter the very structures that condition their behaviour. Structuration theory is, in a sense, a 'reply' to functionalism. Taking its more sophisticated understanding of the social world into account helps us to understand the ways in which top-down policy-making and managerial approaches are over-simple and likely to fail. From this perspective the social world is dynamic and constantly in the process of creation. Structuration is in action on a daily basis. Yet, in contrast to phenomenological perspectives, structuration theory recognizes the importance of structures in conditioning the policy-making and implementation processes.

Technical and Vocational Education Initiative (TVEI): A scheme funded initially by the Department of Employment by which work-related courses are developed in schools and colleges in the context of local TVEI projects. TVEI has now come to an end but was a successful and well-funded project from the mid-1980s to the mid-1990s.

Training and Enterprise Council (TEC) (Local Enterprise Council (LEC) in Scotland): Bodies under the direction of TEED charged with facilitating appropriate vocational education and training for their area. TECs do not provide the training directly but fund other bodies, such as further education colleges, to do so.

Training, Enterprise and Education Directorate (TEED): Formerly Training Agency. Replacement for the Manpower Services Commission (MSC) and responsible for aspects of training both in and beyond school. It is now an integral part of the DfEE.

References

Ainscow, M., Hopkins, D., Southworth, G. and West, M. (1994) *Creating the Conditions for School Improvement*, London: David Fulton.

Alexander, R. (1992a) *Policy and Practice in Primary Education*, London: Routledge.

Alexander, R. (1992b) 'Floodlights, Fanfares and Facile Factors', *The Guardian*, 11 February.

Alexander, R., Rose, J. and Woodhead, C. (1992) *Curriculum Organisation and Classroom Practice in Primary Schools*, London: DES. (The 'Three Wise Men' Report)

Alvesson, M. (2002) *Understanding Organizational Culture*. London: Sage.

Angus, L. (1993) 'The Sociology of School Effectiveness', *British Journal of Sociology of Education*, 14, pp. 333–45.

Apple, M. (1989) *Teachers and Texts*, London: Routledge.

Arnot, M., David, M. and Weiner, G. (1996) *Educational Reforms and Gender Equality in Schools*, Manchester: Equal Opportunities Commission.

Ashworth, P. D. and Saxton, J. (1990) 'On Competence', *Journal of Further and Higher Education*, 14, 2, pp. 3–25.

Ball, C. (1990) *More Means Different*, London: Royal Society of Arts.

Ball, C. (1992) Opening Address. 'The New Renaissance Partnerships in Enterprise Education: an international perspective' 13 July.

Ball, S. J. (1990a) *Politics and Policy Making in Education*, London: Routledge.

Ball, S. J. (1994a) 'Researching Inside the State: Issues in the Interpretation of Elite Interviews', in D. Halpin and B. Troyna (eds), pp. 107–20.

Ball, S. J. (1994b) *Education Reform: A Critical and Post-structural Approach*, Buckingham: Open University Press.

Ball, S. J. (1995) 'Intellectuals or Technicians? The Urgent Role of Theory in Educational Studies', *British Journal of Educational Studies*, 43, pp. 255–71.

Ball, S. J. (1999) 'Labour, Learning and the Economy: a "Policy Sociology" Perspective', *Cambridge Journal of Education*, 29, 2, pp. 195–206.

Ball, S. J. and Shilling, C. (1994) 'Guest Editorial. At the Crossroads: Education Policy Studies', *British Journal of Educational Studies*, 42, 1, pp. 1–5.

Barber, N. (1984) *The Organisation as Curriculum*, unpublished Ph.D. thesis. Wright College, Berkeley.

Barnett, R. (1994) *The Limits of Competence*. Buckingham: Society for Research into Higher Education and Open University Press.

Barrett, S. and Fudge, C. (eds) (1981) *Policy and Action*, London: Methuen.

Becher, T. (1988) 'Principles and Politics: an Interpretative Framework for University Management', in A. Westoby, *Culture and Power in Educational Organizations*, Buckingham: Society for Research into Higher Education and Open University Press, pp. 317–28.

Beckhard, R. and Pritchard, W. (1992) *Changing the Essence: The Art of Creating and Leading Fundamental Change in Organisations*, San Francisco: Jossey Bass.

Bernstein, B. (1970) 'Education Cannot Compensate for Society', *New Society*, 26 February, pp. 344–7.

Bett, M. (ed.) (1999) *Independent Review of Higher Education Pay and Conditions*, London: HMSO (the Bett Report).

Blackburn, R. and Jarman J. (1993) 'Changing Inequalities in Access to British Universities', *Oxford Review of Education*, 19, 2, pp. 197–215.

Blair, T. (1997) 'Why Schools Must Do Better', *The Times*, 7 July, p. 20.

Bleiklie, I. (2000) 'Policy Regimes and Policy Making', in M. Kogan et al. (eds), pp. 53–87.

Bourdieu, P. (1997) 'The Forms of Capital', in A. H. Halsey et al. (eds), pp. 46–58. First published in J. E. Richardson (ed.) (1986) *Handbook of Theory of Research for the Sociology of Education*, Paris: Greenwood Press, pp. 241–58.

Bowe, R., Ball, S. J. and Gewirtz, S. (1994) 'Captured by the Discourse? Issues and Concerns in Researching Parental Choice', *British Journal of Sociology of Education*, 15, 1, pp. 63–78.

Bright, M. (1997) 'Strict New School Day for All Primary Children', *Observer*, 8 June, p. 1.

Brookman, J. (1992) 'Same Song but with a Different Tune', *Times Higher Education Supplement*, 2 October, p. 21.

Bryman, A. (1999) 'Leadership in Organizations', in S. Clegg, C. Hardy, and W. Nord (eds) *Managing Organizations: Current Issues*, London: Sage, pp. 26–42.

Burgess, R. (ed.) (1993) *Educational Research and Evaluation for Policy and Practice?*, London: Falmer Press.

Callaghan, J. (1976) *The Prime Minister's Speech at Ruskin College, Oxford, on Monday 18 October, 1976*, London: DfEE.

Cantor, L., Roberts, I. and Pratley, B. (1995) *A Guide to Further Education in England and Wales*, London: Cassell.

Carter, D. S. G. and O'Neill, M. H. (eds) (1995) *International Perspectives on Educational Reform and Policy Implementation*, London: Falmer Press.

Carter, J. (1997) 'Post-Fordism and the Theorisation of Educational Change: What's in a Name?', *British Journal of the Sociology of Education*, 18, 1, pp. 45–61.

Cerych, L. and Sabatier, P. (1986) *Great Expectations and Mixed Performance*, London: Trentham.

Chitty, C. and Simon, B. (eds) (1993) *Education Answers Back: Critical Responses to Government Policy*, London: Lawrence and Wishart.

Clark, A. (1993) *Diaries*, London: Weidenfeld and Nicolson.

Clark, B. (1972) 'The Organisational Saga in Higher Education', *Administrative Science Quarterly*, 17, pp. 178–83.

Coffield, F. (1999) 'Breaking the Consensus: Lifelong Learning as Social Control', *British Educational Research Journal*, 25, 4, pp. 479–99.

Coffield, F. and Williamson, B. (eds) (1997) *Repositioning Higher Education*, Buckingham: Open University Press/SRHE.

Committee of Vice-Chancellors and Principals (1993) 'Key Points from DFE Announcement on Planned Spending for 1994/5'. Fax to HEIs 30 November 1993, London: CVCP.

Committee on Higher Education (1963) *Higher Education: Report of the Committee Appointed by the Prime Minister under the Chairmanship of Lord Robbins 1961–63* (the Robbins Report), London: HMSO, CMND 2154.

Conservative Research Department (1996) *The Nursery Voucher Scheme: A Brighter Future. Background Briefing for Members of Parliament, Conservative Assocations and Group Leaders*, London: CRD, February.

Coulby, D. and Bash, L. (1991) *Contradiction and Conflict: The 1988 Education Act in Action*, London: Cassell.

Cox, C. B. and Dyson, A. (eds) (1969a) *Fight for Education: A Black Paper*, London: The Critical Quarterly Society.

Cox, C. B. and Dyson, A. (1969b) *Black Paper Two: The Crisis in Education*, London: The Critical Quarterly Society .

Croner (no single date) *The Teacher's Legal Guide*, Kingston-upon-Thames: Croner.

Dale, R. (1985a) *Education, Training and Employment*, Buckingham: Open University Press.

Dale, R. (1985b) 'Technical and Vocational Education Initiative', in Dale (1985a), pp. 41–56.

Dale, R. (1989) *The State and Education Policy*, Buckingham: Open University Press.

Dearing, R. (1997) *Higher Education in the Learning Society*, London: DfEE.

Deem, R. (1996a) 'The School, the Parent, the Banker and the Local Politician: What Can We Learn from the English Experience of Involving Lay People in the Site Based Management of Schools', in C. Pole and R. Chawla-Duggan (1996b).

Deem, R. and Davies, M. (1991) 'Opting Out of Local Authority Control – Using the Education Reform Act to Defend the Comprehensive Ideal:

A Case Study in Educational Policy Implementation', *International Studies in Sociology of Education*, 1, pp. 153–72.

Denzin, N. K. (1983) 'Interpretive Interactionism', in G. Morgan (ed.) *Beyond Method: Strategies for Social Research*, Beverly Hills: Sage.

Denzin, N. (1992) 'Whose Cornerville Is It Anyway?', *Journal of Contemporary Ethnography*, 21, 1, pp. 120–32.

Department for Education (1992) *Education into the Next Century*, London: HMSO.

Department for Education (1994) 'Student numbers in higher education – Great Britain 1982/3 to 1992/3', *Statistical Bulletin*, 13/94, August, London: HMSO.

Department for Education and Employment (1997) *Excellence in Schools*, London: HMSO.

Department of Education and Science (1988) *Advancing A Levels* (the Higginson Report), London: HMSO.

Department of Education and Science (1991a) *Education and Training for the Twenty First Century*, London: HMSO.

Department of Education and Science (1991b) *Higher Education: A New Framework*, London: HMSO, CMND 1541.

Department of Employment (1992) *Progress: Training Credits – a Report on the first 12 months*, London: HMSO.

Egerton, M. and Halsey, A. H. (1993) 'Trends by Social Class and Gender in Access to Higher Education in Britain', *Oxford Review of Education*, 19, 2, pp. 183–96.

Elliott, J. (1991) *Action Research for Educational Change*, Buckingham: Open University Press.

Eraut, M., Steadman, S., Trill, J. and Parkes, J. (1996) *The Assessment of NVQs*, Brighton: University of Sussex Institute of Education.

Etzioni, A. (1967) 'Mixed Scanning: a Third Approach to Decision-making', *Public Administration Review*, 27, 5, pp. 385–92.

Fairclough, N. (2000) *New Labour, New Language?*, London: Routledge.

Finch, J. (1986) *Research and Policy: The Uses of Qualitative Methods in Social and Educational Research*, Lewes: Falmer Press.

Finegold, D., Keep, E., Miliband, D., Raffe, D., Spours, K. and Young, M. (1990) *A British Baccalaureate: Ending the Division Between Education and Training*, Education and Training Paper 1, London: Institute for Public Policy Research.

Fitz, J. and Halpin, D. (1991) 'From "Sketchy Policy" to a "Workable Scheme": The DES and Grant-maintained Schools', *International Studies in Sociology of Education*, 1, pp. 129–51.

Fitz, J., Halpin, D. and Power, S. (1994) 'Implementation Research and Education Policy: Practice and Prospects', *British Journal of Educational Studies*, 42, 1, pp. 53–69.

Fitzgerald, T. H. (1988) 'Can Change in Organizational Culture Really be Managed?', *Organizational Dynamics*, 17, 1, pp. 5–15.

Foucault, M. (1977) *The Archaeology of Knowlege*, London: Tavistock.

Fullan, M. (1991) *The New Meaning of Educational Change*, London: Cassell.

Fullan, M. (1993) *Change Forces*, London: Falmer Press.

Fullan, M. (1999) *Change Forces: The Sequel*, London: Falmer.

Fullan, M. and Hargreaves, A. (1992) *What's Worth Fighting for in Your School?*, Buckingham: Open University Press.

Gamble, A. (1988) *The Free Economy and The Strong State*, London: Macmillan..

Gewirtz, S. and Ozga, J. (1990) 'Partnership, Pluralism and Education Policy: a Reassessment', *Journal of Education Policy*, 5, pp. 37–48.

Gewirtz, S., Ball, S. and Bowe, R. (1995) *Markets, Choice and Equity in Education*, Buckingham: Open University Press.

Ghouri, N. (1998) 'Fantastic News for Teachers', *Times Educational Supplement*, 20 March, p. 16.

Gibson, A. and Asthana, S. (1998) 'School Performance, School Effectiveness and the 1997 White Paper', *Oxford Review of Education*, 24, 2, 195–210.

Gipps, C. and Murphy, P. (1994) *A Fair Test? Assessment, Achievement and Equity*, Buckingham: Open University Press.

Gleeson, D. (1989) *The Paradox of Training*, Buckingham: Open University Press.

Goodson, I. (1990) 'Nations at Risk' and 'National Curriculum', *Politics of Education Association Yearbook*, pp. 219–32.

Government Statistical Office (annually) *Social Trends*, London: HMSO.

Graham, D. with Tytler, D. (1993) *A Lesson For Us All? The Making of the National Curriculum*, London: Routledge.

Green, D. (ed.) (1991) *Empowering the Parents: How to Break the Schools Monopoly*, London: Institute for Economic Affairs.

Hall, G. E. (1995) 'The Local Educational Change Process and Policy Implementation', in D. S. G. Carter and M. H. O'Neill (eds), pp. 101–21.

Hall, V. (1994) *Further Education in the United Kingdom*, London: Collins Education/Staff College.

Halpin, D. and Troyna, B. (eds) (1994) *Researching Education Policy: Ethical and Methodological Issues*, London: Falmer Press.

Halsey, A. H. (1992) *Decline of Donnish Dominion*, Oxford: Oxford University Press.

Halsey, A. H., Lauder, H., Brown, P. and Wells, A. S. (eds) (1997) *Education: Culture, Economy, Society*, Oxford: Oxford University Press.

Ham, C. and Hill, M. (1993) *The Policy Process in the Modern Capitalist State*, Brighton: Wheatsheaf Books, 2nd edition.

Hammersley, M. (ed.) (1993) *Educational Research: Current issues*, Buckingham: Open University Press and Paul Chapman Publishing.

Hammersley, M. (2000) 'The Relevance of Qualitative Research', *Oxford Review of Education*, 26, 3 & 4, pp. 393–405.

Hammersley, M. and Scarth, J. (1993) 'Beware of Wise Men Bearing Gifts: a Case Study of the Misuse of Educational Research', in R. Gomm and P. Woods (eds) *Educational Research in Action*, London: Open University and PCP.

Hargreaves, A. and Reynolds, D. (eds) (1989) *Education Policies: Controversies and Critiques*, Lewes: Falmer Press.

Hargreaves, D. (1996) *Teaching as a Research-based Profession: Possibilities and Prospects*. The Teacher Training Agency Annual Lecture. Mimeo.

Harlen, W. and Malcolm, H. (1997) *Setting and Streaming: A Research Review*, Edinburgh: The Scottish Council for Research in Education.

Hartley, A. (1983) 'Ideology and Organisational Behaviour', *International Studies of Management and Organisation*, 13, 3, pp. 26–7.

Hayter, T. (1997) *Urban Politics*, Nottingham: Spokesman.

Higher Education Statistics Agency (1995) *HESA Data Report: Students in Higher Education Institutions*, July, London: HESA.

Higher Education Statistics Agency (1997) *Students in Higher Education Institutions*, London: HESA.

Higher Education Statistics Agency (2001) *Higher Education Statistics for the UK 1999/2001*, London: HESA.

Hill, D. (1992) 'What the Radical Right is Doing to Teacher Education: a Radical Left Response', *Multicultural Teaching*, 10, 3, pp. 31–4.

Hill, M. (1993) *The Policy Process: A Reader*, Hemel Hempstead: Harvester Wheatsheaf.

Hillgate Group (1987) *The Reform of British Education*, London: Hillgate Group.

Hjern, B. and Hull, C. (1982) 'Implementation Research as Empirical Constitutionalism', *European Journal of Political Research*, 10, 2, pp. 105–16.

Hounsell, D., Martin, E., Needham, G. and Jones, H. (1980) *Educational Information and the Teacher* (British Library Research and Development Report 5505), London: British Library.

Husserl, E. (1931) Ideas, London: Allen and Unwin.

James, M. (1993) 'Evaluation for Policy: Rationality and Political Reality: the Paradigm Case of PRAISE?', in R. Burgess (ed.) (1993), pp. 119–38.

Jary, D. and Parker, M. (1995) The McUniversity: Organization, Management and Academic Subjectivity, *Organization*, 2, 2, pp. 319–38.

Jermier, J. M., Knights, D. and Nord, W. R. (eds) (1994) *Resistance and Power in Organizations*, London: Routledge.

Jones, L. and Moore, R. (1993) 'Education, Competence and the Control of Expertise', *British Journal of the Sociology of Education*, 14, 4, pp. 385–97.

Jordan, G. (1982) 'The Moray Firth Working Party: "Performance" without "Conformance"', *European Journal of Political Research*, 10, 2, p. 117.

Kelly, T. (1983) 'The Historical Evolution of Adult Education in Great Britain', in M. Tight (ed.) *Opportunities for Adult Education*, London: Croom Helm.

Kemmis, S. (1993) 'Action Research', in M. Hammersley (ed.) (1993).

Kerr, C. (1991) 'Is Education Really All that Guilty?', *Education Week*, 27 February, p. 30.

Knight, C. (1990) *The Making of Tory Education Policy in Post-war Britain*, London: Falmer Press.

Kogan, M. (1982) 'Changes in Perspective', *Times Education Supplement*, 15 January, p. 6.

Kogan, M., Bauer, M., Bleiklie, I. and Henkel, M. (2000) *Transforming Higher Education*, London: Jessica Kingsley.

Labour Force Surveys, available at http://www.mimas.ac.uk/surveys/lfs/, last accessed 12 August 2002.

Labour Party (1997) The Politics of the Nursery: Why Nursery Vouchers Are Not the Answer for Our Children, London: Labour Party.

Lauder, H., Jamieson, I. and Wikeley, F. (1998) 'Models of Effective Schools: Limits and Capabilities', in R. Slee, G. Weinder and S. Tomlinson (eds) *School Effectiveness for Whom? Challenges to the School Effectiveness and School Improvement Movements*, London: Falmer Press.

Lawton, D. (1992) *Education and Politics in the 1990s: Conflict or Consensus?*, London: Falmer Press.

Lawton, D. (1994) *The Tory Mind on Education, 1979–94*, London: Falmer Press.

Lee, D., Marsden, D., Rickman, P. and Duncombe, J. (1990) *Scheming for Youth*, Buckingham: Open University Press.

Levin, H. M. and Kelley, C. (1997) 'Can Education Do It Alone?', in A. H. Halsey et al. (eds) (1997). First published in *Economics of Education Review*, 13, 2 (1994), pp. 97–108.

Lindblom, C. E. (1959) 'The Science of "Muddling Through"', *Public Administration*, 19, pp. 79–99.

Lingard, B. and Garrick, B. (1997) 'Producing and Practising Social Justice Policy in Education: a Policy Trajectory Study from Queensland, Australia', Paper presented to the International Sociology of Education Conference, Sheffield, 3–5 January.

Lipsky, M. (1980) *Street Level Bureaucracy: Dilemmas of the Individual in Public Services*, Beverly Hills: Sage.

Maclure, S. (ed.) (1986) *Educational Documents, England and Wales, 1816 to the Present Day*, London: Methuen, 5th edition.

Maclure, S. (1989) *Education Re-formed: A Guide to the Education Reform Act*, London: Hodder and Stoughton, 2nd edition.

McPherson, A. and Raab, C. (1988a) 'Exit, Choice and Loyalty', *Education Policy*, 3, 2, pp. 155–79.

McPherson, A. and Raab, C. (1988b) *Governing Education: A Sociology of Policy since 1945*, Edinburgh: Edinburgh University Press.

McRobbie, A. (1994) *Postmodernism and Popular Culture*, London: Routledge.

Majone, G. and Wildavsky, A. (1978) 'Implementation as Evolution', in H. E. Freeman (ed.) (1978) *Policy Studies Review Annual 2*, Beverly Hills: Sage.

Mandelson, P. and Liddle, R. (1996) *The Blair Revolution*, London: Faber.

Marren, E. and Levacic, R. (1994) 'Senior Management, Classroom Teacher and Governor Responses to Local Management of Schools', *Educational Management and Administration*, 22, 1, pp. 39–53.

Marsh, D. and Rhodes, R. A. W. (1992) *Implementing Thatcherite Policies*, Buckingham: The Society for Research into Higher Education and Open University Press.

Masland, A. T. (1985) 'Organisational Culture in the Study of Higher Education', *Review of Higher Education*, 8, 2, pp. 157–68.

Modood, T. (1993) 'Subtle Shades of Student Distinction', *Times Higher Synthesis*, 16 July, p. iv.

Morris, R., Reid, E. and Fowler, J. (1993) *Education Act 93: A Critical Guide*, London: Association of Metropolitan Authorities.

Mortimore, P. (1997) 'Can Effective Schools Compensate for Society?', in Halsey et al. (eds) (1997).

National Commission on Education (1993) *Learning to Succeed*, London: Heinemann.

National Commission on Education (1995a) *Learning to Succeed After Sixteen*, London: National Commission on Education.

National Commission on Education (1995b) *Learning to Succeed: The Way Ahead*, London: National Commission on Education.

National Commission on Education (1996) *Success Against the Odds: Effective Schools in Disadvantaged Areas*, London: Routledge.

Office for National Statistics (ONS) (2002) *Social Trends 32*, London: ONS.

Office for Population Census and Statistics (OPCS) (1989) *Social Trends 19*, London: HMSO.

Office for Population Census and Statistics (OPCS) (1995) *Social Trends 25*, London: HMSO.

Office for Population Census and Statistics (OPCS) (1997) *Social Trends 27*, London: HMSO.

Office for Population Census and Statistics (OPCS) (2001) *Social Trends 31*, London: HMSO.

Organisation for Economic Co-operation and Development (annually) *Education at a Glance*, Paris: OECD.

Palumbo, D. J. and Calista, D. J. (1990) *Implementation and Policy Process: Opening up the Black Box*, New York and London: Greenwood Press.

Parker, M. (2000) *Organizational Culture and Identity*, London: Sage.

Parlett, M. and Hamilton, D. (1972) 'Evaluation as Illumination: a New Approach to the Study of Innovatory Programmes', reprinted in D. Hamilton, D. Jenkins, C. King, B. Macdonald, and M. Parlett (1977) *Beyond the Numbers Game*, London: Macmillan.

Perkins, D. (1996) 'Minds in the "Hood"', in B. Wilson (ed.) *Constructivist Learning Environments*, Englewood Cliffs: Educational Technology Press, pp. v–viii.

Pettigrew, M. (1994) 'Coming to Terms with Research: the Contract Business', in D. Halpin and B. Troyna (eds), pp. 42–54.

Pole, C. and Chawla-Duggan, R. (eds) (1996a) *Reshaping Education in the 1990's: Perspectives on Primary Schooling*, London: Falmer Press.

Pole, C. and Chawla-Duggan, R. (eds) (1996b) *Reshaping Education in the 1990's: Perspectives on Secondary Schooling*, London: Falmer Press.

Pollitt, C. (1990) *Managerialism and the Public Services: The Anglo-American Experience*, Oxford: Blackwell.

Pollitt, C. (1993) *Managerialism and the Public Services: Cuts or Cultural Change in the 1990s?*, Oxford: Blackwell.

Power, S. and Whitty, G. (1999) 'New Labour's Education Policy: First, Second or Third Way?', *Journal of Education Policy*, 14, 5, 535–46.

Power, S., Halpin, D. and Fitz, J. (1996) 'The Grant Maintained Schools Policy: the English Experience of Educational Self-governance', in C. Pole and R. Chawla-Duggan (eds) (1996b).

Raab, C. D. (1994) 'Where Are We Now? Reflections on the Sociology of Education Policy', in D. Halpin and B. Troyna (eds) (1994), pp. 17–30.

Rand Change Agent Study: Federal Programs Supporting Educational Change, Vol. 1, Berman, P. and McLaughlin, M. W. (1974) *A Model of Educational Change*. R-158911-HEW. (The first of eight volumes published between 1974 and 1978)

Randle, K. and Brady, N. (1997) 'Managerialism and Professionalism in the "Cinderella Service"', *Journal of Vocational Education and Training*, 49, 1, pp. 121–39.

Rein, M. (1983) *From Policy to Practice*, London: Macmillan.

Reynolds, D. and Cuttance, P. (1992) *School Effectiveness: Research, Policy and Practice*, London: Cassell.

Reynolds, J. and Saunders, M. (1987) 'Teacher Responses to Curriculum Policy: Beyond the "Delivery" Metaphor', in J. Calderhead (ed.) (1987) *Exploring Teachers' Thinking*, London: Cassell.

Richards, H. (1993) 'State Tightens Control', *Times Higher Education Supplement*, 3 December, p. 1.

Ritzer, G. (1996) *The McDonaldization of Society: An Investigation into the Changing Character of Contemporary Social Life*, Thousand Oaks: Pine Forge Press.

Robertson, D. (1994) *Choosing to Change*, London: HEQC.

Robertson, D. (1996) 'An Open Letter to Sir Ron Dearing,' paper delivered to the Dilemmas of Mass Higher Education Conference, Staffordshire University, 10–12 April.

Robinson, P. (1996) *Rhetoric and Reality: Britain's New Vocational Qualifications*, London: Centre for Economic Performance.

Robinson, P. (1997) *Literacy, Numeracy and Economic Performance*, London: Centre for Economic Performance.

Sabatier, P. (1986) 'Top-down and Bottom-up Approaches to Policy Implementation Research', *Journal of Public Policy*, 6, pp. 21–48.

Saunders, M. (1986) 'Developing a Large Scale "Local" Evaluation of TVEI: Aspects of the Lancaster Experience', in D. Hopkins (1986) *Evaluating TVEI: Some Methodological Issues*, Cambridge: Cambridge Institute of Education.

Schuller, T. (ed.) (1995) *The Changing University*, Buckingham: Open University Press/SRHE.

Schultz, T. W. (1961) 'Investment in Human Capital', *American Economic Review*, 51, pp. 1–17.

Schutz, A. (1972) *The Phenomenology of the Social World*, London: Heinemann. First published 1932.

Scott, P. (1995) *The Meanings of Mass Higher Education*, Buckingham: Open University Press/SRHE.

Selwyn, N. and Fitz, J. (2001) 'The National Grid for Learning: a Case Study of New Labour Education Policy Making', *Journal of Education Policy*, 16, 2, pp. 127–47.

Senge, P. (1992) *The Fifth Discipline*, New York: Century Publications.

Shiner, M. and Modood, T. (2002) 'Help or Hindrance? Higher Education and the Route to Ethnic Equality', British Journal of Sociology of Education, 23, 2, pp. 209–32.

Taylor, G., Saunders, J. B. and Liell, P. (annually) *The Law of Education*, London: Butterworth.

Taylor, S., Rizvi, F., Lingard, B. and Henry, M. (1997) *Educational Policy and the Politics of Change*, London: Routledge.

Thomson, A. (1997) 'Colleges Too Broke to Educate Properly', *Times Higher Education Supplement*, 7 November, p. 1.

Thomson, A. (2001) 'Does Labour Come Up Smelling of Roses?', *Times Higher Education Supplement, Analysis*, 11 May, pp. 6–7.

Tierney, W. G. (1987) 'Facts and Constructs: Defining Reality in Higher Education Organisations', *Review of Higher Education*, 11, 1, pp. 61–73.

Tooley, J. and Darby, D. (1998) *Educational Research: A Critique*. London: OFSTED.

Trow, M. (1970) 'Reflections on the Transition from Mass to Universal Higher Education', Daedalus. 90, pp. 1–42.

Trow, M. (1994) *Managerialism and the Academic Profession: Quality and Control*, London: QSC.

Trowler, P. (1996) *Investigating Mass Media*, London: Collins Educational.

Trowler, P. and Hinett, K. (1994) 'Implementing the Recording of Achievement in Higher Education', *Capability*, 1, 1, pp. 53–61.

Trowler, P. (2001) 'Captured by the Discourse? The Socially Constitutive Power of New Higher Education Discourse in the UK', *Organization*, 8, 2, 183–201.

Troyna, B. (1994) 'Critical Social Research and Education Policy', *British Journal of Educational Studies*, 42, 1, pp. 70–84.

van Zoonen, L. (1994) *Feminist Media Studies*, London: Sage.

Warner, D. and Palfreyman, D. (2001) *The State of UK Higher Education: Managing Change and Diversity*, Buckingham: Open University Press/SRHE.

Watkins, P. (1994) 'The Fordist/Post-Fordist Debate: the Educational Implications', in J. Kenway (ed.) *Economising Education: The Post-Fordist Directions*, Deakin, Victoria: Deakin University.

Watson, D. (1996) 'Unit Public Funding', Figure 4 of a presentation given at the 'Dilemmas of Mass Higher Education' conference, Staffordshire University, 10–12 April. 1979/80 to 1988/9 figures based on parliamentary question written answer 3 December 1991 for both university and polytechnic data, 1989/90 to 1996/7 data from DFE Departmental Report 1994–5.

Whitty, G. (1997) 'Social Theory and Education Policy: the Legacy of Karl Mannheim', *British Journal of Sociology of Education*, 18, 2, pp. 149–64.

Willmott, H. (1993) 'Strength is Ignorance; Slavery is Freedom: Managing Culture in Modern Organizations', *Journal of Management Studies*, 30, 4, pp. 515–52.

Woods, P. (1992) 'Empowerment through Choice?', *Educational Management and Administration*, 20, 4, pp. 204–10.

Woods, P. (1996) *Researching the Art of Teaching: Ethnography for Educational Use*, London: Routledge.

Woods, P. and Wenham, P. (1995) 'Politics and Pedagogy: a Case Study in Appropriation', *Journal of Education Policy*, 10, 2, pp. 119–41.

Woods, P., Bagley, C. and Glatter, R. (1996) 'Dynamics of Competition', in C. Pole and R. Chawla-Duggan (1996b).

Index